Key Debates in
Health Care

Key Debates in Health Care

Gary Taylor and Helen Hawley

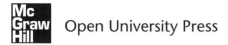 Open University Press

Open University Press
McGraw-Hill Education
McGraw-Hill House
Shoppenhangers Road
Maidenhead
Berkshire
England
SL6 2QL

email: enquiries@openup.co.uk
world wide web: www.openup.co.uk

and Two Penn Plaza, New York, NY 10121-2289, USA

First published 2010

A catalogue record of this book is available from the British Library

ISBN13: 9780335223947 (pb)   9780335223930 (hb)
ISBN10: 033522394X (pb)   0335223931 (hb)

Library of Congress Cataloging-in-Publication Data
CIP data has been applied for

Fictitous names of companies, products, people, characters and/or data that
may be used herein (in case studies or in examples) are not intended to
represent any real individual, company, product, or event.

Typeset by Aptara Inc., India
Printed in the UK by Bell and Bain Ltd., Glasgow.

Mixed Sources

Product group from well-managed
forests and other controlled sources
www.fsc.org Cert no. TT-COC-002769
© 1996 Forest Stewardship Council

FSC

The McGraw·Hill Companies

Contents

Acknowledgements

Without the support and encouragement from friends, colleagues and our families this book would have been impossible to complete. Our thanks go in particular to Mike McManus for showing us the way to make the politics of health accessible and relevant to students training to be health professionals. Alison McCamley has been supportive throughout and we benefit daily from her friendship. We would also like to thank Rachel Crookes at Open University Press for staying with us throughout the process of writing the book and for her sound advice, guidance and good humour. Our reviewers also made a significant contribution to the final shape of this book and we thank them for their comments. Some of the material contained in the book we have previously had published as journal articles. We would like to thank the editor of *Social Policy Journal* for permission to draw upon material from Taylor, G. and Hawley, H. (2004) 'The construction of arguments on the rationing of health care: perspectives from the British broadsheets', *Social Policy Journal*, Volume 3, Number 3, pp. 45–62. Material from Taylor, G. and Hawley, H. (2006) 'Health promotion and the freedom of the individual', *Health Care Analysis*, Volume 14, Number 1, pp. 15–24 has been used with kind permission from Springer Science and Business Media.

Personal thanks and dedications

My thanks go to Karen for discussing many of the issues, commenting upon the draft chapters and for keeping our children happy and well. I would like to dedicate my work in this book to my old family GP Dr Cranston of Kingshurst Birmingham, who stayed up with me night after night in the winter of 1963 and kept me safe.

Gary Taylor

My thanks go to Gavin for his support and understanding during my many hours at the computer and also my parents for their constant faith in my abilities. Thanks also to the Public Health department of NHS Rotherham for giving me a good grounding and frontline experience of a holistic approach to health.

Helen Hawley

Introduction

Chapter Contents

Key questions   The structure of the chapters
The structure of the book   Conclusion

This book is concerned primarily with exploring key debates on the role of the state in the direction and provision of health care and how these debates are reflected in the framing of health policy in a variety of countries. Although its main focus is on the development of health policy in Britain and in the United States, the book also taps into a broader range of international examples. In approaching these debates, we have attempted to capture the flavour of at least some of the conflict and controversy over health care issues. Rather than concentrate upon statistical material on the needs of the various populations or the extent of health care provision in different countries, we have chosen to view the debates in a political context in the belief that recording conflicting views over the aims and processes of health care will help readers to locate themselves in political terms and to think their way through alternative approaches to health care. When we talk about politics, however, we mean it in the broadest of senses. We are interested in capturing and illustrating the importance of different world views. Although political parties and influential politicians will sometimes express these views, they are fortunately not the only source of political insight. Each of us has within our very core something that could be described as political. Consider, for example, the views that we have of each other. Can we trust each other to do what is right? Should the government help those who are unable to help themselves or should every person be responsible for their own welfare? These are political questions. In order to answer these questions, it is not necessary to have a detailed knowledge of political parties or the latest government initiative. Far more important is that we see ourselves in relation to others, as members of the community and as citizens with a range of rights and responsibilities.

Key questions

So what kind of questions should we concern ourselves with? The answer to this depends upon who are the main participants, stakeholders or actors. If we were interested in the internal workings of the National Health Service (NHS) then we would need to identify where power resides in the service, which groups make the decisions and how these decisions are implemented. We have chosen, however, to look in the opposite direction. Rather than looking inwards at an organization like the NHS, we have chosen to look at society. The questions we ask are framed so that we can explore ways to understand, manage and improve the health of each of us. In this book, we will be looking at such questions as:

- Who is responsible for the health of the nation?
- Does this responsibility lie with each individual or is health a social condition for which governments should assume some responsibility?
- Should the state play a major role in the direction and provision of health care or should we rely rather more upon the private sector and upon the increasingly influential voluntary sector?
- Is there a fair way to ration health care?
- To what extent should the state tackle health inequalities?
- Is prevention better than cure?
- What kind of rights should patients have?
- What is the impact of professionalism upon the relationships between different sections of the health care system?

These key questions will provide us with a series of windows into the politics of health policy.

The structure of the book

This book is intended not as a history of health care but as an exploration of ideas and policies on key problems facing modern health care systems. It begins with an examination of different models of health and then moves on to consider eight main debates on issues ranging from the role of the state in the provision of health care to the rights of patients. These debates have been selected in the hope that they will be of some relevance to people training for work in health care. Rather than go into detail on some of the issues that might concern health care managers (such as the mechanisms used to audit quality of provision) we have concentrated on those issues that might resonate more with front-line health care workers. These debates in turn are divided into the three main parts of the book:

- the politics of provision;
- setting priorities;
- patients and health professionals.

In effect, we will be asking who should provide health care, how priorities should be set and in what ways a balance can be achieved between the rights of patients and the interests of the health professions. These key questions represent the spine for the book, upon which the key debates are hung. We will say something about each section by way of introduction.

Part 1 of this study looks at some of the ways in which health care is provided. The key question is, who should provide health care? We will be looking at some of the options open to people when making decisions about their own health care. The main alternatives are dealt with in Chapters 2–4. These alternatives are:

- the state (Chapter 2);
- the private sector (Chapter 3);
- the voluntary sector (Chapter 4).

It will be noted how the balance between these various providers differs considerably across the globe. While some countries have a well-developed system of state health care, others rely to a far greater extent upon the private sector or upon the voluntary sector. We will see, however, that most countries allow for a mix of provision. Even the most committed to state health care, post-war Britain and Sweden for example, allowed some room for the private sector. The opposite also applies. Countries that rely more upon private provision, the United States for example, will still also allow for some state or federal provision to cover those who are unable to attend to their own health care needs.

In Part 2 of the book, we ask how priorities should be set in health care. In the process of researching for this book, we have often come across the assertion that resources for health care are limited and that hard decisions have to be made about where to concentrate investment. While recognizing that the level of this resource can be changed in accordance with the aims and preferences of different governments, we have to acknowledge that there is a multitude of demands upon a health budget and that increasing investment in one thing will often lead to cuts in provision in another area of health care. Instead of trying to take account of all the variables, we have chosen to look at three areas of debate:

- health inequalities (Chapter 5);
- health promotion (Chapter 6);
- rationing (Chapter 7).

These are effectively debates about the allocation of resources within the health system and within state health care in particular. We ask to what extent the state should attempt to alleviate health inequalities, provide health promotion or ration health care. As the previous section shows, the state is not the only provider of health care. The same questions could be asked of the private and voluntary sectors but these questions lie outside the remit of the current volume. Instead, we attempt to understand the priorities set on a theoretical and practical level and to discuss some of the implications for health care professionals.

Part 3 moves away from how priorities are set to questions concerning the rights and obligations of both health care professionals and the patients they serve and we ask to what extent professionalism and patient rights are compatible. This final section contains two chapters:

- patients' rights (Chapter 8);
- professionalism (Chapter 9).

These chapters take us away from the agendas set by governments and allow us to view the relationships between patients and those who work in health care. As with other debates we cover, we are interested in outlining different perspectives on these issues rather than in defending and promoting a single perspective. Conflicting ideas are indeed the lifeblood of this book.

The structure of the chapters

Given the broad scope of the book, we felt that benefits could be gained from adopting a similar format for each of the chapters. Rather than include chapters that vary greatly in the extent to which they use historical examples, contemporary observations, practical illustrations or theoretical insights, we chose to use four main ways to grapple with the issues we cover and to include each of these layers in the chapters included herein. These layers are as follows:

- theoretical perspectives;
- policy developments;
- perspectives of health care professionals;
- health care scenarios.

We argue that each of these will help the reader to appreciate both the broad features of the debates and perhaps some of the subtleties and practical implications of the debates we cover. Let us take a look at each of these in turn.

The first layer deals with theoretical perspectives and will include ideas developed by political theorists, politicians and by some academic commentators. By taking a look at these perspectives, we have an opportunity to examine an issue in the abstract without being pinned down too much to deal with specific policy developments. These ideas are included so as to give the reader an insight into the broad arguments made for and against a particular direction in policy. By taking note of these ideas, it is hoped that readers will be able to locate themselves, even if only provisionally, in terms of some of the alternatives on offer.

In the second layer of the book, we will use examples of policy developments in Britain, the United States and in an assortment of countries. While this is not a book on comparative health policy, comparisons will be made in the hope of illustrating the similarities and differences between the policies developed and implemented in various countries. Although preference will be given to discussing policy developments in English speaking countries like Canada, New Zealand and Australia, comparisons will also be made with parts of the European Union. Once again, we have had to be selective so policy developments in Western Europe (France, Germany, Spain and so on) will tend to feature more than examples from Eastern Europe (for example, Poland, Hungary and Russia). The rationale for this is partly linguistic and partly practical. Access to good quality translations of health policy documents is reasonably limited and we make the assumption (correct or not) that the majority of those who are trained in Britain or the United States will choose to practise either in those countries or in other English speaking nations.

The third layer of the book takes into account the experience and opinions of health care professionals. While there is a wealth of material on policy developments, there is rather less on the opinions and perspectives of professional groups. Professional journals do, however, provide some insight into the views of health care professionals. We have therefore taken a look at a range of journals and concentrated on the views of such groups as nurses, occupational therapists, physiotherapists, doctors and consultants. Although we have not attempted to provide a history or definitive account of these groups and their contribution to key debates in health policy, their views have been included to illustrate the responses of those on the front line of health care delivery and, it is hoped, to reduce some of the distance between those training in health care and the theoretical and policy developments that will shape their working lives. This third layer will be scattered through the book and will feature in some of the boxes we have included. We hope that this will enable the reader to recognize the insight of those actively engaged in the provision of health care as they proceed through the material on theoretical and policy developments.

We have also included a fourth layer that could be defined as health care scenarios. These scenarios are designed to ask the reader to place him or herself into the role of a health care professional and to consider the implications of the debates we cover for those who provide health care. It is by no means our intention to prescribe what health care professionals should do in a certain situation, but to ask the reader to engage in an imaginative exercise. These exercises say in effect that you are a health care professional faced with a certain issue or problem and ask you to consider what you could do in response. It is intended that the reader will take note of the theoretical or policy material included in the book and use these ideas or insights to think their way through the issues and to devise practical solutions. Please be aware that these solutions do not necessarily have to be right or wrong. The scenarios have been included to facilitate understanding of a range of alternatives and to illustrate in a practical way how theoretical and policy developments can be used to inform your own practice.

Conclusion

In writing this book, we have been concerned with finding ways to capture some of the flavour of key theoretical debates on health and health care and to show how these debates can be illuminated with the use of practical examples. It is contended that these debates are relevant to those training to be health professionals and to those attempting to understand the development of policies in different countries. We explore theoretical arguments and policy initiatives in the hope of making a contribution to social and political debates on health care and drawing out the relevance of these debates for health care professionals. While there is a limit to what can be achieved in a single volume, it is hoped that the debates selected will help readers discover for themselves some new ways to understand and appreciate the politics of health care.

1 Health and health policy

Chapter Contents

Tempting as it might be to launch into the key debates, it would seem prudent to pause for a while to consider what we mean by health and health policy. These terms are used throughout the book and are viewed in broadly social and theoretical contexts. What do we mean by this? When we talk about health in its social context we are drawing attention to the myriad of economic, social and cultural factors that influence the way we live and the health we experience. These factors influence who we are and the way we relate to each other. Let us not think of ourselves as having a single social identity, stamped on us for all time. Our identities change throughout our lives, along with our lifestyles and experiences of health. Consider, for example, the elderly couple whose diet is now restricted because of limited income and whose health is fading. Their understanding of health (their own and others) is transformed as a result of their own experiences. They do not need to be categorized. They need to be understood. So what do we mean by a theoretical context? Rather than focus upon the details of empirical research, we are seeking to uncover different approaches to health care. Health policies are consequently seen as illustrating different philosophies of life rather than as dry policy documents. It is contended throughout this volume that our views on the provision of health care often rest upon how we understand the nature of health and upon the way we regard the rights and responsibilities of the individual and the state.

Health

Let us start by taking a look at the nature of health in the broadest of senses. We should begin by recognizing that each one of us will no doubt have a different view of health, partly because we will have different expectations of our own minds and bodies. Somebody who is actively involved in sports will surely have a different view of their health than somebody who is physically frail. The energy levels expected by young people will tend to be very different from those expected by many senior citizens. Parents with young children will often cope for many years with disturbed sleep and might have to make significant adjustments to their lifestyles to reduce the risks of chronic illness. It would seem, moreover, that our views on our own health will change as we move through the various stages of our lives. Because of this, the way we view the possession or absence of good health will probably change over time. There is, in short, a subjective element to the way we conceptualize and experience both health and illness.

Health and social functions

Health could be seen in terms of the ability of the individual to perform their social functions. Different people will have different functions. These might include raising a family, going to work, and tending to our own needs as well as the needs of others. The more our lives connect with the lives of others, the more expectations will be placed upon us. Viewed in one way, our health could be seen in terms of the ability we have or seem to have to fit in and live in accordance with the expectations placed upon us by other members of society. It should be appreciated that health and illness have serious social consequences. Good levels of health help the economic and social system to function effectively, while illness is dysfunctional for both the individual and for society. In order to minimize this dysfunction, the so-called 'sick role' allows people to be sick temporarily. The sick person is exempt from work and many other social obligations but also has a responsibility to seek help and to improve their health (see Aggleton 1990: 9; Daykin 2000: 115). The sick role provides individuals and society with a safety valve. It allows individuals to opt out of social obligations on a temporary basis without in any way minimizing the importance of these obligations. A person might, for example, be suffering from stress as a result of an increased workload. The sick role allows the individual to say 'enough is enough' and to withdraw their labour until they are healthy enough to work.

Scenario 1 Health, social circumstances and the sick role

Kyle is a 20-year-old student from a working-class and ethnic minority background. He is suffering from chronic migraines on a daily basis and is finding it difficult to keep up with his studies and to hold down his job in a local supermarket. He is expected to attend lectures and seminars four days a week and to work in the supermarket two evenings a week and every weekend. Although his parents give him a small allowance, there are limits to what they can afford. Kyle is considering leaving university and his job. He is the only one of his peer group who has gone to university and he believes that they have an easier life claiming unemployment benefits. Kyle is aware, however, that this could have a devastating impact upon his career prospects and that his parents would be disappointed if he chose to abandon his studies.

Questions

You are a health professional working in a university health centre.

1   What kind of advice would you give to Kyle?
2   How do you think his health is being influenced by his social circumstances?
3   To what extent does Kyle need to change his circumstances in order to improve his health?
4   To what extent and in what ways could the 'sick role' help Kyle to deal with the multitude of expectations placed upon him?

Gauging levels of health and illness

Without wishing to make us sound like machines, many people use terms like 'worn out' or 'drained' to describe being in a state of poor health. These terms conjure up an image of a person who for some reason is depleted of energy and is finding it difficult to cope. Blaxter (1990) has used the term 'reserve' to describe the energy we have at our disposal. While this reserve is depleted by health damaging behaviour (like smoking or excessive alcohol consumption) it can be increased through health affirming behaviour (such as exercise or a good diet). Aggleton (1990) has noted that members of the general public, those without any specific bio-medical training, tend to view health in terms of 'the wholeness or the integrity of the person, their inner strength, and their ability to cope' (Aggleton 1990: 13). Health can be seen in fairly functional terms in which we are deemed to be healthy if we can cope in our various roles. This does, however, differ between ages. Older people are far more likely to view their health in terms of their ability to cope and get around, while young people tend to see it more in terms of their general level of fitness (Jones 1994: 3). There are also differences between classes in the way they view health. For example, it has been shown that middle-class women tend to view health in terms of physical fitness and the exercise they take, while working-class women see it as the absence of illness and the ability to 'get through the day' (Aggleton 1990: 14). It is clear that what is seen as healthy for one person is not necessarily the same for another. Anybody who deals with the health of other people needs to be aware of this. The way we describe our own health is unavoidably influenced by the expectations we have of ourselves.

Shifts over time

In addition to there being vast differences in the way that individuals view their own health, the way that health is regarded within our culture will change dramatically over time. The way we see health has changed significantly over the centuries. During the late eighteenth and early nineteenth centuries, various social commentators argued that poor health stemmed from a poor match between the individual and the environment. Lamenting the decline of a rural past, commentators warned about the corrupting influence of modern city living (Davey et al. 1995: 4–6). Poor health was also regarded as quite stylish among some sections of the artistic elite of the late eighteenth and early nineteenth centuries. It became almost fashionable to be thin and pale, to look delicate and ill. The so-called 'tubercular look' (associated with TB) was thought to show distinction and breeding. According to Susan Sontag (1978), the cult of thinness found in women's fashion in the twentieth century (and now beyond) is 'the last stronghold of the metaphors associated with the romanticising of TB in the late eighteenth and early nineteenth centuries' (Sontag 1978: 34). Byron and the Romantic poets and scholars tended to believe that illness made a person interesting and distinctive. Poor physical and mental health gave the impression that the sufferer was sensitive to the core. Those who suffered from TB and had the money to travel became tragic symbols in the work of the Romantics. These people were freed from their daily routines and encouraged to search for meaning. Sontag claims that it allowed the Romantics to retire from the world. Indeed, the Romantics 'invented invalidism as a pretext for leisure, and for dismissing bourgeois obligations in order to live only for one's art' (Sontag 1978: 36). According to this line of thought, illness can have its cultural benefits.

The negative view of health

Health can be viewed negatively (in terms of the absence of something) or positively (as possessing something). If health consists in the absence of disease, people could be seen as being healthy if they do not have a disease. This would be irrespective of how they feel and whether they considered themselves to be healthy. The problem with this view of health is that it assumes that there is a norm for all bodies. It also tends to rely upon a diagnosis being made, most probably by a member of the medical profession. If we are unaware that we have a disease or if this disease has not been diagnosed, does it mean that we are healthy? (see Aggleton 1990: 5–6). Health can also be regarded as the absence of illness. Illness is experienced and consists in the unpleasant feelings that often accompany a disease. The problem with this view of health is that it relies exclusively upon subjective experience (see Aggleton 1990: 7–8). We should also note that illness differs from sickness. Sickness is often calculated according to the number of people seeking medical help and perhaps absence from work. Illness, on the other hand, is about how we feel. We might put up with feeling ill and thus not reach the statistics of those who are deemed to be sick (Jones 1994: 9). While not seeking to minimize the importance of disease, illness and sickness, these notions do not in themselves capture the nature of health. Indeed, these notions do little more than signify the absence of health.

The positive view of health

Health need not only be viewed as the absence of something. Positive views of health emphasize the value of things we possess. In the 1946 constitution of the World Health Organisation, for example, it was declared that health should be seen as 'a state of complete physical, mental and social well-being and not merely the absence of disease or infirmity' (WHO 1946: 1). Although this is an extremely broad definition of health, it does capture the 'positive' dimension of health and alerts us to the need to take into account social as well as individual factors (see also Aggleton 1990: 8 and Jones 1994: 6). This positive view of health also encourages us to find ways to improve or promote good health rather than always think in terms of responding to illness or disease. For those who hold a positive view of health, health is often viewed in a holistic way. Ewles and Simnett (1985), for example, claimed that it is important to acknowledge and give due weight to the emotional, spiritual and societal factors that influence health (Ewles and Simnett 1985: 9). We might of course wish to extend this list to include numerous other things like environmental or psychological factors. Even if the lists provided are incomplete, they do show the importance of looking beyond our ailments to understand the nature of our health.

The view that health consists in something we possess is gaining prominence in policy documents in Britain and elsewhere. The Black Report of 1980 recognized that we need to consider factors other than freedom from pain or discomfort and that we should give due credence to the importance of vigour, well-being and engagement with our communities (Black 1980). Policy documents often recognize that health is not simply the absence of disease but also the presence of physical, mental and emotional well-being (see for example NHS Scotland 2000: 16). It is argued that improving these dimensions of health can enhance quality of life (Scottish Office 1999). Health policy documents in the United States and in New Zealand have stated that good health should be seen in terms of increasing life expectancy and quality of life (US Department of Health and Human Services 2000; Ministry of Health 2006). Policy makers have started to recognize that helping people to come to grips with the nature and importance of well-being can improve levels of health. Rather than see health in terms of the absence of illness, it can be viewed as a dynamic force that can be influenced by circumstances, lifestyle choices, beliefs, culture and environment. It has been argued that quality of life depends upon having the opportunity to make choices and to gain satisfaction from living. Health can indeed be seen as a resource that gives people the ability to manage or change their lives (Health and Welfare Canada 1986). Viewed in this way, the pursuit of good health becomes an aspiration. This is a far cry from the negative view of health with its emphasis upon the problems we experience rather than the potential we have.

The bio-medical model of health

There are two main models that we can use to discuss issues of health. These are known as the bio-medical and the social models of health. The bio-medical model of health gained prominence during the nineteenth century and still holds considerable power. It looks for ways to identify the cause of an illness and seems to assume that illnesses can be classified and treated in an objective way. The individual is indeed objectified and individual health is recorded in case histories. The bio-medical model of health is anchored in provable facts, derived from rigorous procedures. It is concerned with the internal workings of the body and it presumes that our state of health is a biological fact. The model rests upon the belief that it is possible to diagnose a person's health by taking note of the symptoms and that experts are needed to define and manage our health (Armstrong 1986: 47; Gillespie and Gerhardt 1995: 82–3; Senior and Viveash 1998: 10). The bio-medical model of health tends to view health in terms of freedom from a clinically ascertainable disease (Black 1980). One of the main problems with this approach is that it can lead to prioritizing the treatment of short-term acute illnesses rather than long-term chronic conditions. It can likewise serve to funnel resources into expensive cures for diseases while virtually ignoring relatively inexpensive health promotion programmes (US Department of Health and Human Services 2003). As the bio-medical model of health deals with identifiable illnesses, it is felt that it is possible to identify and gauge the results of medical intervention.

There are a number of problems associated with the bio-medical view of health. In particular, it rests upon a limited view of knowledge and it subjects too many aspects of life to medical measurements. The bio-medical model assumes that medical knowledge is scientific and objective. This knowledge is thought to enable those who possess it to understand the human body, the causes of an illness and the benefits of intervention. What this fails to take into account is that this form of medical knowledge has been created by a small minority and is merely one interpretation of health and illness (Senior and Viveash 1998: 13). It could be argued that members of the medical profession have a vested interest in promoting an overly medical view of life and in diagnosing normal changes in the life cycle as periods of illness. With the backing of drug companies and limited by the time available for consultation, medics often rely upon using drugs to treat rather than concentrate upon promoting better health and preventing illness (Senior and Viveash 1998: 14–15). This bio-medical model of health tends to categorize people according to the illnesses they experience.

The social model of health

The social model of health rejects the neutrality and scientific pretensions of the bio-medical model and regards reliance upon the scientific method as merely one way to measure health. The social model of health acknowledges that health and illness are created socially and that the health we experience relates to the way society is organized. According to this view, health has an historical, cultural and social context and cannot be understood unless we appreciate this (Gillespie and Gerhardt 1995: 82–3). Whereas people who believe that we are isolated and autonomous individuals might believe that it is possible to change our circumstances and make rational choices about our lives regardless of our backgrounds, those who believe that we are social creatures and that our health has a social context understand that any autonomy we might have can be undermined by poor health (Black and Mooney 2002: 197). Government agencies have recognized that health has a social context and that a range of social factors will influence the health we experience. Policy makers in Scotland recognize that our physical and mental well-being will be influenced by the work we do, our housing, the education we receive and the environment in which we live (Scottish Office 1999). In Canada, it has been acknowledged that biology, lifestyle, health care organizations and our social and physical environments will have significant impacts upon our health (Health and Welfare Canada 1986). The Department of Health in Northern Ireland has argued that poor health is often caused and made worse by poverty, unemployment, low educational attainment, poor sense of community, environment, conditions under which we live and work and the lifestyles we lead (DHSSPS 2002: 38). It would appear from the above that the social model of health has an increasing amount of support among policy makers.

There might, of course, be a cynical reason for this. The social model of health allows far more room for policy makers to intervene and tinker with the nation's health. By tracing our health to social factors, they attempt to convince us that we need an active state to intervene to regulate this broader social context and that this intervention will help to improve general levels of health. Even if we agree with this general assertion, it is important that we are aware of its political dimension. Campaigns designed to heighten awareness of the social context of health are political in themselves in that they often challenge the power base of the medical hierarchy. As we will see when dealing with professionalism (Chapter 9), nurses have been particularly important in promoting a patient-centred approach to health care that takes into account the broader social context. We should be aware, moreover, that the conflict between the bio-medical and social models of health is played out at times within teams of health care workers and that those engaged in health care may well be able to locate themselves in one camp or another (see Box 1.1). Although the social model of health is appealing to those who wish to use the state to reform the economic and social system, it is likely to be seen as less attractive to those who want to free the individual from the influence of an interventionist and intrusive state.

Box 1.1   Health professionals and the social model of health

As we have seen the social model of health recognizes that our health will be influenced by our social circumstances. This model of health is gaining greater credence among health care professionals. Doctors have become increasingly aware of the importance of social, economic and cultural factors in the development of conditions and in tackling health problems. This has allowed doctors to understand and respond to the impact of adverse social conditions upon the health of their patients (see Willems et al. 2005). The nursing profession has a long tradition of holistic practice and it is noted that an increasing number of nursing departments have moved away from a bio-medical approach and have adopted a holistic approach to health care (see Thompson and Hammer 2007). A distinction is sometimes drawn between 'cure' and 'care'. Although we might associate 'cure' with physicians and 'care' with nurses, it has been argued that these two values should be viewed along a continuum and that all health care workers should aspire to combine 'cure' and 'care' in their practice. Rather than attempt to set a balance between 'cure' and 'care' in the abstract, commentators have argued that the balance should shift along the continuum depending upon the particular needs of each patient. This would mean that the relative importance of 'cure' and 'care' would vary between cases (see Baumann et al. 1998).

The bio-medical model of disability

One of the key ways to understand the differences between the bio-medical and social models of health is to examine how these models can be applied to a specific area. Consider, for example, different approaches to disability. The bio-medical model of disability regards it as an illness. It portrays people with disabilities as problems and attempts to exert control over their lives. Using the bio-medical model, it is assumed that if we could treat all forms of illness we could do away with disability. This rests upon and reinforces the belief that disabled people are both ill and inferior (Marks 1999: 59 and Drake 1999: 10–11). Traditional views of disability portray people with disabilities as having medical problems that place a limit upon what they can do (BMA 2007: 3). It has been argued that the bio-medical model of disability pays far too much attention to the 'impairments' of people with disabilities and that this creates obstacles to their full participation in society. It is believed by some that society's attitude and reaction to impairments and illness creates real barriers for disabled people (Scottish Parliament 2006). Bury (1996) argues that the medical model of disability is used to protect the existing system. By treating people with disabilities as sick and in need of medical intervention, it gives enormous power to medical practitioners. Disabled activists claim that the disabled rather than medical practitioners should be in charge of the rehabilitation process (Bury 1996: 26). It should be appreciated that the bio-medical view of disability creates an extremely narrow and potentially dangerous view of disability. Apart from anything else, it disempowers people with disabilities and seems to leave them at the mercy of medical judgement rather than as citizens with a range of different needs.

The social model of disability

The social model of disability attempts to undermine this imbalance of power and advance the view that disability is not a medical problem but one stemming from material and cultural forces. Indeed, the idea of disability could be seen as oppressive and one that can be used to erect barriers to sections of the community. The idea of disability could be seen as something imposed from above on top of any impairment. It might also serve to exclude some sections of the community from full participation in economic, political and social life (Barnes and Mercer 1996: 6–7). It has been argued that disability should be distinguished from impairment and ill-health and be seen as 'disadvantage experienced by an individual . . . resulting from barriers to independent living or educational, employment or other opportunities . . . that impact on people with impairments and/or ill health' (Prime Ministers Strategy Unit 2005: 8). According to the BMA (2007), people are not disabled by impairments but by society and by the way that activities and opportunities are organized. People with disabilities are urged to take control of their situation and challenge the disabling barriers created by society (BMA 2007: 3–4). This view of disability recognizes that social attitudes need to be challenged and that social facilities and opportunities need to be made accessible to people with diverse needs.

The more we view disability as an illness, the more likely we are to find ways to quarantine those with disabilities from those without.

The social model of disability sets out to undermine self-blame and self-hate among people with disabilities and urges us to value the abilities rather than the disabilities of people. People with disabilities can often find themselves isolated from the mainstream of society. It has been noted that up to 20 per cent of disabled people find themselves cut off from activities they enjoy and that they are more likely than people without disabilities to live in poverty, have fewer educational qualifications, to be out of work and be subject to prejudice and abuse (Prime Ministers Strategy Unit 2005: 5–6). Governments across the world have come to recognize the importance of empowering people with disabilities. In the United States, the Department of Health and Human Services has argued that attention should be placed upon improving the relationship between people with disabilities and their environments (US Department of Health and Human Services 2005: v). In Canada, approaches to disability stress the importance of facilitating independent living, social networks and inclusion in the life of the community (Health Canada 2007). The Ministry of Health in New Zealand approaches disability as part of its commitment to human rights. It is argued that we must tackle the barriers that disable people and that human rights must apply to all people (Ministry of Health 2001: 3). The social model of disability and of health in general does indeed encourage us to challenge oppression and discrimination on a number of levels and to recognize that the labels handed out by the medical establishment can be dangerous and can be used to marginalize significant sections of the community.

Scenario 2   Models of disability

John is a 25-year-old man who has had to use a wheelchair since his motor cycle accident in his teens. Following his accident, he lost his partner and his job. His social circle has shrunk and he has become increasingly depressed. John's physical health has also deteriorated. He has almost doubled his body weight and he now smokes habitually.

Questions

You are a health care professional working in a local day centre, which John uses two days a week.

1   Why is it important to distinguish between John's illness and his disability?
2   What could be done to improve John's health?

Health policy

Having looked at some of the general features of health and illness, we now move on to consider the broad dimensions of health policy. Once again, the aim is to create some foundations rather than to define all forms of health policy or to provide a comprehensive list of everything health policies embrace. Health policy is one of the means by which the state can intervene to direct or provide for the health care needs of the nation. As we will see, the extent of this intervention differs greatly between countries and the question of how far the state should intervene is subject to a great deal of debate. What could be called the social policy perspective on health is concerned primarily with the role of the state in the provision of health care. It looks at what the state does, how policies are made, the historical development of state provision and at the various demands for reform. It seeks to determine the appropriate role of the state, the way in which health is organized and combines such disciplines as ethics, politics and economics (Lloyd 2001: 164–5). It should be appreciated at the outset that health policy is often developed as part of a broad package of social policies. If the government assumes some responsibility for tackling poor health, it makes sense that this is done in conjunction with other social policy initiatives in such areas as housing, unemployment, poverty reduction and education. In Ireland, for example, health policy is closely linked with other policy areas such as economic development, employment and urban regeneration (DHSSPS 2002). It is often the case that agencies or ministries are called upon to work together to deal with health problems. In New Zealand, for example, the Ministry of Health and the Ministry of Social Development work together on those social projects that have a bearing on health (Ministry of Health 2006). It must surely be the case that treating health in isolation would fail to give due attention to the broader social factors influencing our health. For example, somebody might be suffering from depression as a result of being made redundant and feeling trapped in poor housing or a deprived area. We would suggest that no amount of medication could improve matters long-term for this person and that providing them with opportunities for meaningful work and personal development would probably have a greater impact.

The importance of partnerships

Although the state is one of the main players in the development of health policy, we should recognize that health care is often formulated and delivered through partnerships with a variety of groups in the community. The Department of Health in Britain recognizes and embraces partnerships. In the consultation exercise that fed into *Choosing Health* (2006b), the Department of Health worked with key stakeholders from the NHS, local government, the business community, the media, faith groups and the voluntary sector (DH 2006b). The NHS in Scotland is involved in a series of important partnerships, where the government and community organizations work together to identify the origins and possible solutions to poverty, poor educational attainment and poor health (NHS Scotland 2000: 4). In Northern Ireland, partnerships have been created between government departments, public bodies, local communities, voluntary groups and district councils (DHSSPS 2002: 7). In the United States, the Department of Health and Human Services has a number of strategic partnerships with non-federal organizations, especially in the field of health promotion. The structure of these partnerships allow for the Department of Health and Human Services to coordinate community initiatives rather than assume direct responsibility for providing health care (US Department of Health and Human Services 2007a). This illustrates, among other things, how the development of health policy and the delivery of health initiatives often involve a process of negotiation with key stakeholders, each of which may well have its own agenda to defend and to promote. This can make the development of health policy a rather messy affair.

Implementing health policy

It might be tempting to believe that governments with a clear majority of seats in their parliament have a free hand in making policy and in implementing their ideas as intended. But the barriers to making and implementing policy are numerous. Policy is not necessarily made in a methodical manner, where problems are identified objectively and alternative solutions are considered, monitored and evaluated. More often than not, policy is made in an incremental way by a variety of groups vying for influence and support (Palfrey 2000: 33–6). Not all groups, of course, have equal power. Within the British health system, for example, the British Medical Association (which represents the interests of doctors) will tend to have a greater influence on health policy than the Royal College of Nursing, which represents the interests of nurses (see Cameron 1999: 123–4 and 132–3). This does not mean that political and medical elites will always have their own way, as policies are not always implemented in the way intended by policy makers. Policies generally have to be implemented by people lower down the hierarchy than those who made the policies. Although policy makers might want their policies to be implemented as designed, this would rely upon a rigid command structure in which objectives and tasks were clearly defined and in which the support of the main actors (doctors, nurses, managers, etc.) for the policy initiatives of the organization could be guaranteed. What this fails to take into account is the existence of diversity within organizations and that the consequences of attempting to apply a policy are not always clear at the outset. It has been noted that a considerable amount of discretion is used in implementing policy, especially by the so-called 'street level bureaucrats' who tend to be the human face of the organization because of their contact with the public. These street level bureaucrats include nurses in health care and teachers in education (Palfrey 2000: 42–6). Governments might be able to set the agenda and design policy frameworks, but this does not guarantee success in initiating change. Without the support of key stakeholders, policies can be sabotaged.

Conclusion

This is a book about health rather than about illness. We do not in any detailed way account for the rise or prevalence of certain illnesses nor are we interested in concentrating upon the weaknesses of any particular health care system. Instead, we want to make sense of health and of at least some of the issues that policy makers have to face. By comparing different health care systems, it is hoped that we can come to understand possible solutions and, when coupled with some understanding of theoretical perspectives, start to think about the implications of different approaches to health policy. We recognize at the outset that health care should be concerned not only with repairing us when we are ill but also with capturing our hearts and minds. Throughout the volume you will see signs of a commitment to finding ways to address social problems and to enhance health and well-being. The issues we discuss will allow us to investigate the relationship between health and society and the impact of the economic and social climate upon health and the availability of health care. We will see that there is rarely if ever only one solution and we hope that we have left enough room in the debates for you to develop your own perspectives on health care and upon the responsibilities of both the government and the individual. By delving into the social and political context of health care, we hope to show how each of us has the power to make a difference, however small, to the health and well-being of our communities.

PART 1
THE POLITICS OF PROVISION

2   The state

Chapter Contents

It makes sense for us to begin our account by taking a look at the state. One of our key aims is to outline some of the conflicting views of how far the state should intervene in health care. This will provide an important framework for the book and a context for the debates that follow. We begin with some questions:

- Can we trust the state?
- Does it represent the common good?
- Should the state be responsible for providing health care for all citizens?
- Should we be responsible for our own health and health care?

These questions can be explored by taking a look at a range of theoretical perspectives and policy developments concerning the role of the state in the provision and direction of health care. What is meant by the state does of course differ across the international system. In Britain, the term state generally refers to the national government and to the institutions it uses to exercise power. In the United States, the term is more often used to refer to the various state governments that are united on a national level by the federal government. The term state is used in this volume to refer to the workings of national government. When specific references are made to the system in the United States, the term federal government will be used instead. Many countries in the developed world allow some room for state provision of health care. Sometimes this is provided out of principle. As we will see, access to health care can be viewed as a fundamental human right that should be guaranteed by the state. If this is the case, then the state should have a role in directing health care in the nation and (in order to enhance its directive powers and to prevent abuses in the system) perhaps some degree of ownership of the health service. This does, of course, raise issues about the right of individuals to tend to their own health needs and to set up as independent practitioners. The status of private practice in those economic and social systems heavily dependent upon state intervention is contentious and will be discussed in greater detail in Chapter 3. For now it is worth bearing in mind that for some people private practice is viewed in a positive light and state intervention is regarded with suspicion. These critics of state intervention are often willing to allow the state to furnish health care in the last resort only, such as when individuals are incapable of providing for themselves. According to this perspective, state intervention in the provision of health care might be expedient but never preferable.

Theoretical perspectives

When assessing to what extent the state should be involved in health care, we are confronted by vibrant political debates that draw upon some of the key political ideologies in the Western political tradition. There are many different ideologies. They include liberalism, conservatism, socialism, feminism and so on. Ideologies are constructed by theorists and practitioners to make sense of the social and political systems and to suggest possible ways to either protect or transform these systems. They often rest upon clear assumptions about the nature of humanity and the motives that dominate our actions. Are we isolated individuals or members of a community? Are we capable of living in a cooperative way or are we naturally competitive? To what extent should we be free to dispose of our income as we wish? Is taxation a form of theft? These are the kind of questions that appear in social and political discourse, which is concerned not only with what the government does but also with the relationship between the government, the individual and the community. The state is granted various powers and functions, by both theorists and practitioners, because of assumptions about what we are capable of doing by ourselves. If all people were capable of looking after their own economic and social welfare, there would be little need for the government to direct economic and social affairs. Divisions of opinion on whether the state should intervene in health care should be seen in the context of these broader debates about the relationship between the individual and the state. We are interested in exploring not only different views on the desirability or otherwise of state involvement in health care but also how these views fit into broader philosophies of life.

Arguments for state intervention

Those who argue in favour of the state playing a major part in the provision and/or direction of health care often do so in the belief that health should be viewed in its social context. Rather than see us as isolated individuals responsible for our own health care, it could be argued that our economic, social and physical environments influence the health we experience. For example, somebody who works in a factory on night shifts may well experience a different state of health to somebody who works in an office during the day. Somebody who is long-term unemployed is less likely to be able to access the sporting facilities available to those who can afford the fees required for gym membership. As we will see when we discuss health inequalities (see Chapter 5), there are numerous ways in which sections of the community can suffer from poor health as a result of their broader economic and social circumstances. The question remains, however: is the state under any obligation to do anything about this? For advocates of state intervention, if health is a social product then the state does have at least some responsibility to tend to the health needs of the nation.

Egalitarian
State involvement in health care could be seen as a means by which the state can enhance equality or at least compensate for some of the inequalities apparent under a capitalist system. Under a capitalist system, based upon the private ownership of the means of production and the pursuit of profit, there will undoubtedly be winners and losers. This inequality could be viewed as necessary to inspire people to succeed economically. Critics of capitalism will point out, however, that the state could do something to humanize capitalism and to make it a less brutal system for those on low incomes. Consider, for example, the views of Labour Party politicians during the 1950s. Inspired by visions of social democracy, they believed that the state could be used to usher in a peaceful transition to socialism in which the state would take a more active role in managing the economic and social system (see Taylor 2007). Aneurin Bevan regarded the NHS in England and Wales as a fine example of what could be done through collective action (Bevan 1952). For Tony Crosland (1957), it was valued because it could encourage the development of social unity and equality. Egalitarians believe in the essential equality of human beings and argue that policies should be developed to enable people to become as equal as possible. Because of this, they claim that society should aim to establish equal health status and grant equal access to health care. This would necessarily involve giving more resources to disadvantaged sections of society in the hope of raising their level and their life chances (see Hoedemaekers and Dekkers

2003: 327–30). As we shall see, the belief that the state should use its power to reduce inequalities has played an important part in the development of state health care in many countries.

Civic

The argument in favour of state intervention in health care does not have to be tied to a broader programme of economic and social change. State intervention could be defended and advanced on the grounds that it is essential for our maintenance as individuals. Charles Kennedy, the former leader of the Liberal Democrats in Britain, has argued that equal access to health care is a necessary condition for individual freedom (Kennedy 2001: 104). Allowing the state a significant role in health care might also be defended on the grounds that it serves democracy and that it can encourage citizens to be more active in their communities. State involvement in social provision is sometimes supported because it enhances fellowship and allows us to participate more fully in public life. In the Netherlands, for example, it is argued that citizens have a collective responsibility to provide health care for all. All citizens contribute towards the cost of health care and trust that the health care system will be there when they need it (Houtepen and Muelen 2000: 362–6). This civic argument differs from the egalitarian argument in that it seems more concerned with making the current system work than with pushing for fundamental political change. The civic approach attempts to appeal to our sense of civic responsibility rather than to any fundamental reservations we might have over the value of capitalism.

Social

The case for state intervention in health care might also take note of how individuals are tied to others in society and how this creates a series of responsibilities towards each other. The wealth and health possessed by any individual is rarely, if ever, the result of individual effort alone. Many factors influence our general welfare and we should be willing to acknowledge that our need for health care is unpredictable and will no doubt change considerably at different stages in our lives. If this is the case, it would make sense for us to pool our risks and share the costs of health care. In this way, we will benefit both individually and collectively. It is clear, however, that this argument rests upon seeing each other as neighbours and as moral beings (see Ashcroft et al. 2000). The social argument outlined above could be accommodated into many different political ideologies. It is compatible with social democratic ideas but also with some forms of both liberalism and conservatism. One of the strengths of the social argument is that it illustrates that what is good for the community is also good for the individual. If we accept that we are connected in this way and that individuals benefit from collective endeavours, then a case for state intervention in health care can be made with relative ease.

The egalitarian, civic and social arguments outlined above are by no means mutually exclusive. For example, somebody who is attracted to egalitarian views might also want to see a society in which our civic ties and responsibilities are strengthened and they might recognize moreover that it makes sense to be egalitarian in outlook because of the ways in which we are dependent upon each other. Rather than seeing these arguments as separate and independent of each other, we should recognize that they are connected. It is far more a matter of emphasis than of having to choose one over another. Arguments for state intervention in health care will tend to view health in its social context and share the belief that in some way or another we are social animals with responsibilities towards each other. For those who view society in this way, the state is seen as having the potential to tend to the health of the nation and in so doing help to create a society based upon cooperation rather than upon competition. These arguments are devised to appeal to our sense of community and to our ideals. The selfishness of which we are all capable is relegated in importance and we are left with a view of what could be if only society was organized in a sensible and perhaps ethical manner. For supporters of state intervention, it would be foolish to rely upon individuals to usher in fundamental social change. A far more reliable approach recognizes that the state can be used to invest in the economic and social systems and to coordinate activities in the interests of all rather than leave the individual to pursue their own interests regardless of their impact upon society.

Scenario 3   State intervention

Derek is a 57-year-old ex-miner who has lived and worked in the same mining town all his life. He has been forced to take early retirement as he suffers from Chronic Obstructive Pulmonary Disease (COPD) and therefore has severe respiratory difficulties. This condition is primarily caused by his working history, but is exacerbated by his continued smoking. The state plays a major role in Derek's health care. He has access to full NHS support for his COPD and attends a specialist community group for rehabilitation (he is given free transportation to get there). After rehabilitation he will continue to receive care. His COPD is seen as a lifelong condition which requires long term management. He also receives support from a smoking cessation advisor to help him give up smoking and is given free Nicotine Replacement Therapy (NRT).

Questions

1   To what extent do you believe that the state has an obligation to treat Derek?
2   Do you think that the state should provide all the services described above?

Arguments against state intervention

Arguments against state intervention in health care tend to proceed from the assumption that health is a possession for which we are responsible as individuals. If we are responsible for our own health, then the state has no duty or obligation to tend to our health needs and we should be willing and expect to pay for our own health care. The same line of reasoning can be applied to a number of our economic and social needs. If we are unemployed, it might be regarded as our responsibility to find work rather than rely upon government benefits. The same logic would urge us to invest in the education of our children on the grounds that they will benefit from this investment in the future. This perspective on life sees us all as isolated individuals and gives each person the freedom to choose how to spend their own income. The alternative, in which the government taxes citizens and spends money on their behalf, is considered fundamentally flawed.

Neo-liberalism

Neo-liberals in particular believe that the state should avoid being too entangled in the direct provision of health care and leave most of it to private practice. Neo-liberalism is a relatively new political ideology. It started to develop in the years immediately after the Second World War when many liberals began to look towards the state to alleviate economic and social problems. For neo-liberals, the spirit of classical liberalism needs to be revived. Neo-liberals defend the capitalist system and the values it perpetuates. The neo-liberal world is one based upon individual achievement and on keeping the government as small and as unobtrusive as possible (see Taylor 2007). Neo-liberals argue that we should be made responsible for our own health and health care. Hayek (1960), for example, was extremely critical of state intervention in health care. In his view, such intervention would give the state too much power over the life of the individual and he believed that such power could be used to coerce citizens. Hayek believed also that the state ownership and direction of health care failed to capture the significance of the personal bonds between health care providers and their patients. Health care was seen as a personal matter; something between the individual and the health care professional rather than as something that should or could be mediated by the state. It should be noted that this line of argument tends to assume that under the direction of the state, health care becomes impersonal and devoid of compassion. Standardized and publicly funded, health care provided by the state is viewed as inferior to private health care (see Chapter 3) and as an affront to individual freedom.

Relieving the tax burden

Some of those who argue against state intervention in the provision of health care have pointed out that such intervention will invariably increase the tax burden upon society (see Green 1995). It could be argued that taxation not only deprives individuals of resources but also the freedom to make decisions about how to dispose of their own income. Reducing taxation could therefore be seen as a move consistent with individual freedom. This economic argument appears in a variety of guises. It might be said, for example, that the publicly funded NHS in Britain ignores the rights of consumers and allows the government the freedom to deduct money for the service without specifying in advance the amount it would take and the services that this money would buy. Green (1995) suggests that the NHS should be privatized and that a well designed insurance system would benefit the poor far more than the present system of public funding. Viewed from an economic perspective, the state might seem to have too much discretionary power to decide how to spend taxpayers' money. This argument feeds on the aversion that many people feel towards paying taxes and to losing control over how this money is spent. We should always remember that the bulk of the money spent by the government, especially in the developed world, is raised through taxing its citizens. This can be through income tax, a tax levied on consumer goods (VAT in Britain) or through some form of corporation taxes on businesses. Those who want to reduce levels of taxation, for whatever reason, will often have to find ways to cut into what the government does and find alternative ways to finance public ventures. Arguments in favour of privatizing the NHS can be seen in this light.

It is supposed that a neo-liberal society would have minimal government intervention and relatively low tax bills. Those who argue in this way believe it is natural for individuals to compete rather than to cooperate. Arguments against state intervention in health care frequently urge us to assume more responsibilities for our own health and welfare. The more responsibility we assume for ourselves, the less tax we can expect to pay and the more control we can expect to have over our own incomes. A case could be made with relative ease for individuals to have the freedom to determine the level of care or provision they want. Although this will be limited by the ability to pay, there are numerous ways that individuals can make provision for their own health care including payment of a fee for each service or through a system of private insurance. For those who believe the state should withdraw or keep out of health care provision, individuals must be allowed to make decisions about their health care rather than be restricted to what the state is willing or able to provide. Although this might appear to be a rather harsh philosophy, in that it could leave the poor with relatively little protection, it tends to appeal to those who want more control over their own income. It is a philosophy of life anchored firmly in self-interest rather than one that seeks to maximize the social good.

Scenario 4   Individual responsibility

Let us return to Derek, who suffers from COPD but continues to smoke. The state plays a very limited role in Derek's life. He has been provided with some support through his pension from the National Coal Board. He is given basic support to help him manage his own COPD, but because he has chosen to smoke (even though he understands it aggravates his COPD) he is given little support to help him give up smoking. His doctor has suggested that he attends a self-help group and has advised him to purchase NRT.

Questions

You are a health professional working in a community setting:

1   To what extent should Derek be responsible for funding his own health care?
2   By continuing to smoke, does Derek fail to fulfil his obligations/responsibilities as a patient?

The third way

There would appear to be little common ground between the arguments for and against state intervention in health care. For those who argue in favour of state intervention, the state is seen as the guardian of the social good or common interest. We are asked to recognize that we are connected to others in society and that our long-term interests are unavoidably linked with those of the collective. Given this, we are urged to pool our skills, resources and finances to build a system that guarantees all citizens decent social provision. For those who are critical of the state, this does nothing more that fuel a bureaucratic machine that seems intent on redistributing wealth and resources away from those who are economically successful by rewarding those who are deemed unable to attend to their own needs. These arguments for and against state intervention in health care by no means cover all participants in the debate but they can be regarded as the opposing factions in many political debates on health and welfare. Many people, however, are willing to pick and mix from both streams of thought in an attempt to devise what could be described as a third way. This has been expressed politically to varying degrees by President Clinton in the United States, Tony Blair in Britain and Chancellor Schroder in Germany (see Taylor 2007). For those who believe in the third way, state intervention and individual responsibility are not mutually exclusive.

The third way and the state

Advocates of the third way recognize that health is influenced by social factors so the state should have some part to play in the provision and direction of health care. It has been argued that old-style social democracy gives too much power to a centralized state and that neo-liberals place too much faith in market forces. In an attempt to avoid the problems of too much state control and of the chaos of market forces, the Blair government in Britain advanced a compromise in which the state established national standards to be adhered to while the provision of health care would rest upon creating partnerships between the state, the private sector and the voluntary sector (DH 2003a; Blair 2003). This approach allows the state to have a major role in the direction of health care without being too entangled in the provision of services. There are undoubtedly advantages to adopting this position. In particular, it allows the state to keep an eye on the public provision of heath care and to set targets for health care providers while at the same time it can remain distant from the day to day problems and shortcomings of the service. This sense of distance might be particularly important during times of cuts in provision and in light of it being unlikely the state will ever be able to provide a fully comprehensive service. As we will see in Part 2 of the book (Chapters 5–7), there are competing demands for resources and, in the context of a limited budget, it is necessary to prioritize some services over others.

Mixed economy of care

The third way involves the creation and maintenance of a mixed economy of care. Rather than rely primarily on the state, the private sector or the voluntary sector, it is believed that these providers can work in tandem as long as the health care they provide is coordinated by the state. For those who believe in a third way, it is important that we take into account and make use of a variety of providers of health care. It could be argued that the quality of the health care provided is far more important than who provides this care. It is noted, moreover, that health problems are often connected to other social problems. The Blair government, for example, recognized that if the government wants to eradicate poor health, it must also address other social problems and dedicate resources to fight social exclusion. For this reason, health policy in Britain is tied to a range of policy areas including housing, employment, crime prevention and so on (see Blair 2003; DH 2003a; Taylor 2007). This theoretical perspective recognizes the interconnected dimensions of health, health care and our broader welfare.

*   *   *

The theoretical perspectives outlined above provide us with a platform to discuss health policy in a variety of countries and will be developed throughout the volume when we move on to discuss both theoretical and policy developments on a range of issues. The social democratic view calls upon the state to assume direct control over health care provision. The neo-liberal view wants to free individuals from state control and rely to a far greater extent upon private health care. The third way, finally, seeks to take something from both approaches to create a hybrid system. There are clearly many other theoretical perspectives that could have been considered. Marxists, feminists, the greens, anarchists, fascists and so on all have views on using the state in health and welfare services. Some of these ideas will no doubt feature in the debates contained in this volume. The social democratic, neo-liberal and third way approaches, however, provide us with a rough framework to consider some of the key policy developments in recent times and we maintain that these approaches have been particularly important in determining to what extent the state should have a role in the ownership and direction of health care in a variety of countries.

Scenario 5 The third way

Think back to Derek in the first two scenarios. What kind of health care could he receive under a third way approach? Derek receives a combination of care. He is given support and health care by the state, but has also been encouraged to join a self-management programme. He has attended a specialist community group for rehabilitation but is now urged to make his own travel arrangements. Here he is encouraged to meet with others to discuss how best to deal with his health problems. He has also been encouraged to attend a community-based exercise programme, for which he will have to pay a small fee. He is given support to help him give up smoking and receives his NRT on prescription (for which he has to pay a standard fee).

Questions

You are a health professional in Derek's community:

1   To what extent should Derek be responsible for managing his own condition?
2   Does the state provide Derek with a sufficient amount of health care?
3   How does the third way approach differ from the other two approaches?

Policy developments

If we are to scrutinize the role of the state in the provision of health care, it is important that we take note not only of theoretical perspectives but also of debates around policy. Theoretical perspectives can provide us with an insight into the way the state is viewed in the abstract. They allow us to think about the rights and responsibilities of individuals in relation to the state and to consider to what extent individuals should be responsible for maintaining and paying for their own health care. It is clear, however, that debates around policy developments show us how governments seek to increase or shrink the role of the state in the provision of health care. Taking a look at these debates and developments will provide us with specific examples of how the state has intervened or withdrawn from health care and what has prompted these changes in government policy. As always, the examples provided will necessarily be selective. It is hoped, however, that they will provide us with a flavour of some of the debate surrounding key policy developments in Britain and beyond.

Britain

The state has been involved in health care in Britain for over a century. Although there were key stages in the development of state activity in health care, we should bear in mind that state involvement developed in an incremental fashion. State intervention in health matters was initially spurred on by the belief that such intervention would help to 'civilize' the masses. This argument was put forward in Britain during the nineteenth century when the government responded to the rapid spread of infectious diseases in urban areas by establishing new public health authorities. Improving health standards was deemed necessary for the moral development of society (see Blakemore 1998: 45–7). In Britain, the National Insurance Act of 1911 introduced a system of sickness benefit in which doctors would act as independent contractors, but would be paid for by the state. Sickness benefit was available to all who were in paid employment and who paid their national insurance stamp (Hill 1997: 20). Those who worked were covered by National Insurance, but as these tended to be men it meant that the majority of women and all children were excluded from cover. Women often had to treat themselves and resort to their own remedies. Only in emergencies would a doctor be called to treat the majority of women and children (Channel 4 1998). This system remained in place until the Second World War, when the need for health care expanded rapidly and plans were made for increasing and maintaining the role of the state in the provision of health care. Here is a clear illustration of the ways in which the state becomes involved in health care. State intervention was born of necessity and stemmed in many ways from increased demands upon the health service during times of war. Having pledged resources to health care, it would have been difficult for post-war governments to back out of their commitments.

Labour policies

A social democratic Labour government in 1948 established the NHS in England and Wales. This government was motivated by egalitarian principles. It effectively nationalized health care and made it free at the point of delivery and financed through general taxation. This was justified on the grounds that the nationalization of health care would make it a more efficient and rational system and that it was essential to ensure equal treatment for all (Klein 2001: 15). All branches of health care were covered until the 1950s, when charges were introduced for dentists and opticians (Taylor 1999: 106). The NHS was founded with the aim of promoting equity of access to health care for people in England and Wales. This means that:

- disadvantaged sections of society should not have inferior care;
- resources should be allocated according to need;
- attempts should be made to encourage those whose health is poor to access the services available.

(DH 1998)

The Labour Party has remained committed to the state having some role in the provision of health care since establishing the NHS. In the period 1945–1979 the Labour Party was motivated by social democratic ideals and it focussed on the positive benefits of state intervention in health care. For example, the Labour Party (1950) acknowledged in its election manifesto that all sections of the community (including the middle classes) benefited greatly from the introduction of the NHS. In the 1960s, the Labour Party (1964) attacked plans to charge for visiting the doctor and called for the abolition of prescription charges. By the end of the 1970s, public opinion was turning against the Labour Party and its reliance upon running a large and expensive public sector. The Labour Party remained convinced however of the importance of the NHS. The Labour Party (1979) believed that the Conservatives planned to create a two-tiered health system consisting in a premium service for those who take out private cover and an inferior service for the rest of the population. It was claimed that the Conservatives wanted to increase the range of services for which the payment of a fee was required while Labour claimed to be working towards the abolition of all charges in the NHS. For the Labour Party, the state needed to do more rather than less.

Conservative policies

The pressure to reduce the role of the state in the provision of health care came from the Conservative Party. Although the Conservative Party had been critical of the idea of the NHS (Conservative Party 1945), it did lend its support to state involvement in health care when it returned to office during the 1950s, 1960s and during the early 1970s (see Klein 2001). By the end of the 1970s, however, the Conservative Party was spearheading neo-liberal policies in Britain. The Conservative governments of the 1980s and 1990s saw health as an individual possession and tended to blame the victims of poor health for their afflictions. It was argued that the working class in particular must change their lifestyles, improve their diets and give up smoking. This lifestyle explanation for poor health served to obscure problems arising from socio-economic conditions (Abercrombie and Warde 2000: 487–8). The Conservatives also believed that the NHS needed to be made more efficient. Mrs Thatcher attacked the view that this was detrimental to patient care and maintained that efficiency and compassion are compatible (Thatcher 1984). The Conservative Party (1987) acknowledged that although the NHS is not a business, it should still be run in a business-like manner in which waste is avoided, efficiency is advanced and managers are encouraged to be innovative and enterprising. Business techniques were therefore introduced into the NHS.

Conservative governments during the 1980s sought to maintain state funding of the health service but transform the way that the service was run by introducing managerial techniques and an internal market. It was believed that consensus management, which involves trying to find agreement between various sections of the health system, should be abolished and replaced by a new hierarchal system run by designated managers. These reforms were thought necessary to tame the bureaucratic features of the NHS and to transform the health system from one run in the interests of health care professionals to one that was more responsive to the needs of patients (Alcock et al. 2000: 196; Allsop 1995: 98–123; Watts 1994: 92; Budge et al. 1998: 617). This move towards managerialism was extended during the late 1980s by the introduction of the internal market. It was thought that internal competition between the various branches of the NHS would make it a more efficient, economical and accountable system. Under the internal market, the government continued to fund the NHS but its various sections became purchasers and providers of services. The internal market made hospitals into financially independent trusts. The income they received depended upon the services they provided. General practitioners also gained control over their own budgets. The money they received depended upon the number of patients on their books. Part of this budget would then be used to purchase health care from hospitals that would compete for business by attempting to offer the most cost-effective treatment (Alcock 1996: 70–1; BBC2 1996b; Allsop 1995: 110–11; Glennerster 2000: 187). In many ways, the Conservative governments of the 1980s and

1990s approached the NHS like a publicly owned business rather than like a traditional public service. Greater autonomy was given to health managers, whose position came to rely upon succeeding in the market place rather than simply administering a public service. Under these conditions, the balance of power within the health service was dramatically altered. This is something that we will return to when we discuss professionalism in a later chapter.

New labour and the third way

When the Labour Party returned to office in 1997, attempts were made to steer the NHS away from its preoccupation with business and towards new community partnerships. Inspired by the thought of devising a third way between social democracy and neo-liberalism, the newly elected Labour government of 1997 criticized the internal market for shifting resources away from patients and towards the administrative costs incurred through competition between sections of the NHS. It was argued that this had a disastrous effect upon the priorities pursued in the NHS. In particular, it created instability and forced managers to think primarily about surviving in the short-term rather than in developing the service for the long-term. The health service was also forced to function without reference to the real needs of the community. Members of the public were apparently unable to access reliable information about the future plans of health care providers in their areas, mainly because these plans were subject to constant change as sections of the health system competed with each other for funding. The Labour government declared that the internal market was to be replaced by a system of 'integrated care' based upon partnerships between health care providers. It was argued that collaboration should replace the competitive approach favoured by the Conservative government. This was envisaged to rely upon piecemeal change rather than a complete upheaval of the existing system of health care (see DH 1997).

One of the key ways in which the Labour government sought to create a new system of integrated care was to increase investment and innovations in primary care. Each primary care group covers a population of about 100,000 people and is given a fixed budget to tend to the health needs of their patients. Health Improvement Programmes have been set up to draw in a variety of local partners and Health Action Zones to look into inequalities in health. Partnerships have been created between the health service, the voluntary sector and local government. The Labour government consulted a broad range of professional groups when developing its policies on health. It was keen to establish a broad consensus and encourage cooperation between professional groups. Health trusts were also instructed to democratize their procedures, hold their meetings in public and involve the public in management committees (DH 2000; Glennerster 2000: 217–18; North 2001: 133–5). Primary care was emphasized in the hope of relieving the pressure on hospitals. If people could be treated before ailments became too severe, then savings might be made and the NHS could become more responsive to the needs of local communities. New multidisciplinary teams were created to deal with a wider range of health care problems affecting people in the community (see Box 2.1). It was argued that these teams would be better placed to understand the health needs of local people and it was assumed that patients would feel less alienated by having local primary care trusts taking care of them rather than having to travel to hospitals in other areas (see DH 2003a).

Box 2.1   The changing roles of health professionals

It is recognized increasingly that health problems can have a variety of dimensions and that poor health can often be traced to a range of social circumstances. Moves toward providing health care through multidisciplinary teams create new opportunities for health professionals. For the Labour government in Britain, the newly decentralized health care system was seen as beneficial for health professionals. The decentralization of power was thought to extend the freedom of health care workers to develop their own methods to support patients and it has been argued that a more decentralized system provides greater opportunities for staff to take on new roles (DH 2006a: 28). Here is a clear example of how policy changes, driven by a desire to alter the way the state supports health care, can have a direct impact upon health care professionals and provide opportunities for career development.

For the Labour government, especially under Tony Blair, it was important to decentralize the provision of health care. The state would still have ultimate power to determine the priorities for public funds. National Service Frameworks were introduced to focus attention on a range of medical problems and new regulatory bodies were established including the National Institute for Clinical Excellence (NICE) and the Commission for Health Improvement (CHI). These aimed to identify priorities and prescribe standards to be attained (see North 2001: 133). The policies were designed to energize the NHS. For the Labour governments of 1997 onwards, the NHS is worth maintaining and reforming to meet the needs of the modern era. The Brown government of 2008 onwards argued that access to decent health care should be seen as a moral right and should remain funded through taxation and free to those who need it (DH 2008d). As we will see in subsequent chapters, the NHS faces a number of serious problems related to the resources at its disposal and the priorities it chooses to pursue. It is certainly the case that health professionals have some reservations about the sustainability of the current service (see Box 2.2).

Box 2.2   Health professionals and the NHS

Arguments in support of the NHS will often focus upon its contribution to society and its enhancement of our social rights. We should, however, also consider the opinions and insights of health care professionals.

Physicians have pointed out that state health care systems, especially in Britain and in Canada, often lack suitable facilities and experience extreme shortages in suitably qualified health workers (Blendon et al. 2001: 242).

It is recognized that the resources available in NHS hospitals are often limited and that hospital facilities in particular are usually drab and uninspiring. Supporters of the NHS point out, however, that quality of care is often of an excellent standard (see Smith 2005: 478).

For others, the NHS has systemic weaknesses that make it unsuited to the modern age. According to one consultant physician, the NHS is no longer efficient or viable. While it might have suited the conditions facing many people in post-war Britain, it is argued that this does not mean that it is still of significant value. In particular, the consultant argued that the NHS:

- provides a low level of service;
- is expensive;
- requires doctors to be 'jacks of all trades' rather than specialists;
- expects doctors to be social workers rather than medics;
- should be replaced by an insurance-based system that puts the needs of the patient first.

(see Goldby 2002)

We should recognize, however, that many of these reservations about the quality of care available could also be viewed as pleas for further investment either from the state or from the private sector. If the NHS is failing to keep up with innovations in care and with the expectations of patients, this does not necessarily mean that state health care in itself is fundamentally flawed.

The United States

Governments in the United States tend to have relatively little to do with the provision of health care. The main political parties in the United States appear to regard federal intervention in social provision as something that might have to happen if private initiatives fail to provide sufficient cover rather than as something to be supported out of principle. Free market and libertarian ideas are firmly entrenched within the American political system. This can be seen in particular since the late 1970s when interventionist policies were deemed to be too expensive and governments looked for ways to reduce federal expenditure (Bailey 2002). Because of this, individuals are more often than not called upon to provide for their own health care rather than to rely upon government provision. The Federal government does, however, have some role in the provision of health care in the United States. It is recognized by many mainstream political parties that not all people are able to fund their own health care and that the government should provide at least some semblance of a safety net.

Democratic policies

The Democratic Party has done a fair amount to increase the role of the state in health care. Lyndon Johnson, the Democratic President between 1963 and 1970, introduced major health care reforms as part of his radical social policy agenda known collectively as the 'Great Society'. Medicare was introduced as a form of social security for the elderly and Medicaid was put in place to assist the poor. This programme led to a rapid increase in federal support for health care. Indeed, the federal health care annual budget increased from $4 billion to $14 billion (Ginsburg 1992: 131; Clarke and Fox Piven 2001: 30–1). Democrats have continued to support state intervention in health care, though since the 1990s the influence of 'third way' thinking is apparent in the approach to health policy taken by the Democratic Party. Leading Democrats like Bill Clinton and Al Gore have argued in support of expanding health coverage to a greater number of citizens (see Campbell and Rockman 1996; American Presidency Project 2000; Clarke and Fox Piven 2001; Linder and Rosenau 2002) while acknowledging that a system of cost sharing was needed to take into account the responsibility each of us has for our own health (Democratic Leadership Council 1991: 9). The Obama government increased the number of health centres across America with the intention of providing further services for those with little or no health insurance (Seblius 2009). Public investment in children's health was increased to relieve the pressure on low-income families and Medicaid was extended to cover those who were moving from welfare benefits to paid employment (US Department of Health and Human Services 2009). For Democrats in the United States, federal government intervention is often viewed favourably as long as it does not destabilize individual freedom or responsibility for oneself.

Republican policies

The Republicans are rather less convinced of the benefits to be derived from federal government involvement in health care. President Eisenhower wanted to establish federal aid for health care but found that fellow Republicans condemned his plans for giving too much power to the government (Damms 2002). Richard Nixon favoured a mixture of public and private provision. He believed that people in work should be covered by a system of health insurance and that the government should have a limited role to help those who are not covered by private insurance (Nixon 1971). During the years of the Reagan government, restrictions were made on Medicare and Medicaid programmes and these restrictions pushed an increasing number of people towards employment-based insurance schemes (Clarke and Fox Piven 2001; Moroney and Krysik 1998: 129). George Bush senior was adamant that the government should as far as possible keep out of health care (American Presidency Project 1992). For the Republicans, the state is seen as a potential drain upon individual initiative and should therefore be excluded as far as possible from a direct role in providing health care and many other welfare services. This approach to health care has left many citizens without sufficient health cover and is of concern to many health professionals (see Box 2.3).

Box 2.3   Health professionals and the American system

Health professionals who have worked in Britain and the United States have pointed out that the American system is often far more advanced in terms of the facilities available to staff (Walder 2003: 497). Where the American system does not fare so well is in the extent to which it can provide for all citizens. Physicians have argued that the main problems facing the American health care system stem from the high costs of care, which means that many people go without proper care and without the medication they need (Blendon et al. 2001: 242). According to some health professionals, government provision of health care is far from adequate. In the state of Oregon, for example, there are only 10,000 places available in the state health care plan but there are over 90,000 hoping to gain access to this health care. It is estimated that over half a million people in Oregon are without health insurance. For John Drake, the director of a community clinic in Portland Oregon, government provision of health care in the United States is in need of fundamental reform (see Mirchandani 2008). When judging the relative merits of different health care systems it is important that we are clear about the criteria we apply. Are superior facilities more important than equality of access to health care? If the state does provide health care, does it need to provide it to the standards we expect from the private sector? It might be that the private sector can provide better facilities (in terms of buildings and décor) and be more able to focus upon the expressed needs and wishes of the consumer, but is this proof of a superior service? The way that each of us views different health care systems will depend upon the values we hold and upon the way we want to finance health care.

International comparisons

The role of the state in the provision of health care differs greatly across the globe. Although the level of state intervention in any one country will change over time, it is still possible to identify those countries that are willing to use the state and those that look to limit state involvement. As we have seen, the state has a significant role in health care provision in Britain but rather less so in the United States. Other health systems that rely heavily upon state intervention include the Swedish and the Canadian systems. The main alternative approach rests upon the payment of insurance premiums. Although there is considerable variation in how this works, insurance-based health care is prevalent in Japan, Hong Kong, Germany and Switzerland.

State health care

The state has had a major role in health care provision in Sweden, where health care is guaranteed to all citizens because of a common commitment to notions of equality and to a belief that all people are of equal value (see Holm et al. 1999: 321–4). For many years, the Swedish health system was held up as a great example of what the state could do and of the apparent success of social democratic policies. For much of the period following the Second World War, the main political parties in Sweden were in favour of extensive state involvement in the social and economic life of the nation. The extent to which Swedish governments were willing to intervene in health care, however, changed quite drastically in the late 1980s and early 1990s when neo-liberal ideas started to gain more credence. Rationing of some health care services was introduced in the 1980s and in the early 1990s market principles were applied to the allocation of health care resources (Gould 1993: 189–95). Although the Swedish government reduced state involvement in health care, Sweden remains one of the best examples of a publicly funded health care system.

Canada has a system of publicly funded health care in which all Canadian citizens have access to primary, secondary and dental care. Although federal government sets guidelines for the system, public health care in Canada is administered on a local or territorial basis (CHO 2007). Government involvement in the provision of health care in Canada was developed in an incremental way. Rather than the federal government taking the lead, public health care was introduced in the provinces and this effectively pushed the federal government to assume some responsibility for the nation's health. In 1947, the government in the province of Saskatchewan introduced universal access to hospital health care. This system was also introduced in the provinces of Alberta and British Columbia in 1949. Not until 1957 did the federal government agree to pay towards the costs of some hospital and diagnostic services incurred in the Canadian provinces. This in turn encouraged other areas in Canada to introduce public health care and by the early 1960s all provinces in Canada had some form of public health care provision (Health Canada 2005: 10). It has been argued that a system of public health care has significant economic benefits. If employers are relieved of any obligation to provide health care packages for their workers, this can lead to lower labour costs and thereby sharpen the competitive edge of businesses in the international economic system. This in turn is considered to be an important factor in the relative success of the Canadian economy (see Health Canada 2005: 12). We can see in this the view that the public funding and provision of health care can benefit a country in a variety of ways. Rather than see public health care as a drain upon the nation's resources, defenders of state intervention may well see public health care as a long-term investment in the health of all citizens and as a necessary foundation for sustained economic and social development.

Insurance-based systems

Whereas the British, Swedish and Canadian health systems grant to the state significant powers to raise money for health care in an effort to advance the public good, other systems depend more upon individuals assuming responsibility for their own health care and upon people taking out their own health insurance. This way of financing health care has been used in many countries. The Japanese state offers limited health services. The system is funded mainly through occupational and national insurance (administered locally), though patients still have to find anywhere between 20 and 30 per cent of the bill when they visit doctors (Uzuhashi 2001: 110). In Hong Kong, private practice dominates primary care but the bulk of secondary care is provided in publicly-funded hospitals (Health and Medical Development Advisory Committee 2005a). In Hong Kong there is a tendency to see individuals as being responsible for their own health and well-being. Although the Hong Kong government is willing to subsidize health care for those who are impoverished, it wants individuals to make contributions towards the costs of their health care (Health and Medical Development Advisory Committee 2005b). If individuals are responsible for their own health care, then the state has no real obligation to run an extensive health system. Where the state does intervene, this can be presented as a form of state charity or something of a last resort for those who are unable to provide for themselves.

Not all insurance-based systems are anchored in an individualist ethos. Indeed, the state can intervene by establishing a compulsory insurance system. Systems of compulsory social insurance operate in both Germany and Switzerland. In Germany, conservatives introduced the heath insurance system in the hope of undermining the appeal of socialism. This system accounts for approximately two thirds of German health spending. In Switzerland, health insurance companies are subsidized through taxation but they have no public guarantee against losses. Many of them operate on a not-for-profit basis and are prevented from diversifying into other forms of insurance cover (Theurl 1999: 332–49). Under systems of social insurance, people have rights to health care and these rights go beyond the limitations of their individual insurance portfolio. It should be recognized that systems based purely upon individual contributions cannot guarantee equity of access or social justice and that a health system financed primarily through individual insurance premiums is unlikely to appeal to those who believe that the state has obligations to its citizens in the field of health care. Public health care in Spain, for example, was boosted by the General Law of Public Health Care of 1986 which transformed the Spanish system from one based upon individual insurance premiums to one based upon access to all citizens regardless of the amount they have contributed in insurance payments (Embassy of Spain 1995). When determining who should provide health care we are indeed often left with a choice between conflicting political positions. One of these positions places priority on the rights of the collective and the other upon what the individual can afford.

Conclusion

We now have a platform anchored upon divergent views on the possible roles of the state in the provision and direction of health care. Three main theoretical perspectives have been outlined. Each of these has been important in the development of health policy in a variety of countries. Social democratic views draw our attention to the social context of health and to the argument that access to health care should be regarded as one of our key social rights. These ideas have been important in the development of health care in Britain and Sweden, especially in the period 1945–1979. During this period, the state was given extensive powers to provide and direct health care and to improve the health of the nation. Under this system, state health care is provided in the majority of cases free of charge and health professionals became public servants responding to health needs rather than to market forces. In the period 1979 onwards, however, neo-liberal ideas challenged the state control of health care. Neo-liberals attempted to divert our attention away from the social context of health and towards our responsibilities for our own state of health and for the costs of our own health care. The state was effectively pulled away from the direct management of health care and health systems were transformed with the assistance of managerial techniques imported from the private sector. These ideas have influenced health policy in Britain, the United States and in many other parts of the world. Under a neo-liberal system, health professionals shed the role of public servant and are expected to be far more aware of market forces and the economics of health care provision. This approach is deemed to be too extreme by many who argue that there must be a third way between social democracy and neo-liberalism. Under the third way, health is viewed once again in its social context but the state is given the task of co-ordinating the activities of a variety of providers of health care rather than running the health system itself. Health professionals are drawn into multi-disciplinary teams working in the community to fight social exclusion. These perspectives and approaches to policy are of course subject to change and to development. They represent, however, some of the building blocks for health policy and will certainly appear in various guises throughout this volume. We now turn to look towards some of the alternatives to state provision.

3   The private sector

Chapter Contents

If we are not willing to trust the state to organize and provide health care, then we need to identify some alternatives. As we have seen already, those who argue against the state having a major role in the provision of health care are often (though not always) supporters of the private sector. This chapter looks at political debates over the value of the private sector. It is always worth beginning with some questions in mind. These questions can help us to structure our thoughts and to guide us through our reading.

- So do we need a private sector in health care?
- To what extent does the pursuit of profit hinder the provision of care?
- Are private practice and public service mutually exclusive?
- What, if anything, should be done to regulate private health care?

The answer to many of these questions depends to a great extent upon the way we view our own responsibilities as individuals and upon the way we see the alternatives. For those who believe that we should be responsible for our own state of health and our own health care, the private sector is perfectly suited to provide health care. If we are responsible for our own health and we damage that state of health, then surely we must be responsible for paying for our own health care. But what about those who cannot afford private health care? What should be done to tend to their health care needs? It may well be a question of choosing from which foundation you look at these issues. Should the private sector be there to supplement a state health system or should a state health system be there to cater for those who are unable to access private health care? As we shall see, both approaches have been adopted in different countries.

The private sector includes independent practitioners and those who supply the public sector with a vast array of products and services. It is increasingly important in health care provision in Britain and has a central position in health systems across the world. The relative importance of private provision differs of course between nations. In Britain, about 10 per cent of health care spending is in the private sector. In Italy, the figure is approximately 23.5 per cent and approximately 33 per cent in the United States (Blank and Burau 2004). It has been noted that approximately seven million people in Britain are covered by private health insurance and that an extra third of a million pay for private operations every year (Browne and Young 2002: 10). Many of us consume goods and services from the private sector even if we are unaware of it.

There are a number of ways in which the private sector is involved in the provision of health care. Since the 1980s, the number of people in Britain choosing to make at least some use of private health care has risen considerably. Care for the elderly is increasingly in private hands, as witnessed by the growth of private nursing homes (Ranade 1997). Long waiting lists and extreme discomfort will often push those who can afford it in the direction of private health care for certain types of treatment. Hip replacements and operations for varicose veins and hernias are particularly lucrative areas for the private sector (Baggott 2004: 140). There has also been a marked increase in the participation of private firms in the NHS. Domestic, catering and laundry services are often provided by private businesses (Renade 1997). The NHS indeed spends most of its budget on goods and services it purchases from the private sector. Pharmaceutical companies swallow a considerable amount of this money (Baggott 2004: 148–9). Of course, sometimes we have little choice. The private sector might be the only provider of the service we require. It was estimated during the 1990s that as many as one in seven British people used private health care to gain access to a broad range of alternative remedies (Ackers and Abbott 1996: 122). We should remember finally that private practice often exists alongside public service, even in state medical systems like the NHS. Consultants can treat their own private patients in NHS hospitals. The NHS indeed is the largest supplier of private health care in Britain (Baggott 2004: 149). We must therefore proceed with care. When discussing private health care, we need to recognize that although there are visible signs of private clinics and hospitals, the extent of private sector provision is often concealed. The public and the private do not always exist in two different locations. They can share the same buildings and the same staff. What separates these two sectors is who pays the bill. For the public sector it is more often than not the taxpayer. For the private sector, it is individuals and/or their insurance companies.

Theoretical perspectives

In the previous chapter we looked at the argument that the state should intervene in health care and saw that it often rests upon assumptions about the nature of health, its socio-economic context and upon the belief that the state can do some good by taking control of the nation's health service. We also saw that the state is sometimes criticized for being unnecessarily intrusive and individuals are asked to make their own decisions about the health care they want and are willing to pay for. Those who are critical of state provision are, almost by default, supporters of the private sector. For those who are in favour of the state, the private sector can be seen as superfluous and in some cases morally inferior. When looking at arguments for and against private sector involvement in health care, we are engaged in debates about the rights and responsibilities of individuals and the extent of our obligations towards each other.

Arguments in support of the private sector

Arguments in favour of private health care often stem from distinct views about the level of responsibility we have for the maintenance and improvement of our own health. If health is seen as an individual possession, then it makes sense that each of us should assume some responsibility for maintaining this possession in reasonable condition. The suggestion that individuals should be responsible for their own health is sometimes used to counter the view that we have an absolute right to health care and to suggest we should be responsible not only for the state of our own health but also for financing our own health care (see Hoedemaekers and Dekkers 2003: 326–7). Supporters of private health care tend to concentrate less on our supposed social rights (to health care, education, housing and so on) and make rather more of the freedom we have as individuals to make decisions about our health and about the level of health care we want to access. The money spent by an individual on private health care could indeed be viewed as a form of investment in oneself and as such has little to do with the government.

The problems with state health care
The case for private health care often draws comparisons with what is offered by the state. Indeed, the private sector is sometimes represented as superior

to the public sector. In a report written for the right wing think tank, the Adam Smith Institute, Browne and Young (2002) claimed that the NHS is 'a politically controlled state monopoly that is institutionally unresponsive to the needs of the patient' (Browne and Young 2002: 4). Health commentators have been keen to point out that the case for private health care is often simultaneously a critique of the public sector. Julian Le Grand, for example, claims that the case for private provision of health care often rests upon criticisms of existing state provision. In particular, it is felt that public provision is too slow to adapt to new technologies and pays too little attention to the needs and desires of patients. Conversely, the private sector is considered better at eliminating waste, responding to the needs of patients and adapting to technological change (Le Grand 2001: 4). While the public sector is viewed as cumbersome and out-dated, the private sector is seen as forward-looking and better suited to respond to the diverse needs of patients. This view of the private sector would seem to have some support from health professionals (see Box 3.1).

Box 3.1   Health professionals support for private health care

There is no reason to believe that health professionals in the state sector would have negative views towards the private sector. Although nursing unions have often been critical of the private sector, many of their members have in recent years been turning towards the private sector for treatment. For example, Mary Brown who works as a nursing instructor for the NHS claims that quality and innovation is often lacking in the NHS and the private sector can usually provide a more speedy and convenient service. Peggy Prior, a branch secretary for the Royal College of Nursing, has argued that although many nurses feel uncomfortable about going private the NHS is failing to provide a suitable service (see Hastings and Fraser 2001). For these health professionals, it is apparent that their hearts remain with the NHS but they feel they are forced to access private health care because of the limitations of what the state can offer. We should not be surprised by this. Health care workers in the state sector know (perhaps better than other people) the limitations of the current service. Increasingly, they will also have greater knowledge and access to the private sector. Divisions between the two sectors are far from rigid and the more the state places limits upon the health care it is willing to finance, the more health care workers will become aware of the importance of the private sector for certain procedures. The importance and visibility of the private sector increases each time there are cuts in state health care.

The economic benefits of private health care

Supporters of private health care have also noted its economic benefits. The private health sector could be seen to expand choice for patients and in so doing force private health care providers to 'raise their game' and to be innovative in the treatment and care they offer. By encouraging entrepreneurial skills and product development, the economy might be seen to benefit (Propper et al. 2006: 8). Private health care might also be beneficial in encouraging prudence. For example, in 1992 the parliament of Guernsey debated plans to scrap free hospital care and require all residents to take out private health insurance. In support of this, the President of the Guernsey Board of Health claimed that 'in those communities where patients are billed and made aware of the costs, it has been demonstrated that people act responsibly and utilise the service when necessary, but not indiscriminately' (Chilcott cited in Brindle 1992: 21). The economic benefits of private health care could therefore be seen in terms of motivating the providers and encouraging patients to be a little more frugal in the resources they consume. These arguments tend to imply that under a system of state health care providers have little incentive to improve the service and the patients have little incentive to prevent them from being wasteful in consuming resources regardless of real need.

Scenario 6   Illustration of the potential benefits of the private sector

Let us consider the potential benefits of the private sector by making use of a scenario. Edna is an 85-year-old woman who is housebound after a recent hip replacement operation and needs help bathing to ensure she does not get an infection. She has health insurance and can use this to pay for her own private health care package. This gives her an opportunity to choose the type of support she needs, when she needs it and who provides it.

Questions

You are a health care worker attached to an out-patient department in a state hospital. You are aware of the limited resources available for care following operations:

1   How would you advise Edna to proceed with her rehabilitation?
2   Should more resources be made available through state health care for post-operative care or should this be left for individuals to finance?

Arguments against the private sector

One of the arguments against private health care is that it depletes state health care systems of resources and takes advantage of the foundations created by government investment. There are a number of ways this might occur. Baggott (2004) points out that by allowing consultants to continue private practice in the NHS, this could distract them from caring for NHS patients. The private sector also benefits greatly from the training and staff development provided by the public sector. Given this, it would appear that the private sector grants to itself the right to profit from state investment without having to assume any direct responsibility for improving the health of the nation. Critics may well point out that private practice lives like a parasite upon the public sector. Rather than standing alone as independent contractors, it could be seen that the private sector derives a lot of its business from the referrals of state health care providers and does relatively little to train the next generation of health care professionals. Without the assistance of the public sector, the private sector might find it difficult to survive.

The problem of injustice

The existence of private health care could be seen to undermine social solidarity and extend social injustice. It has been noted that private health care providers 'rate poorly on equity considerations because they link the availability of treatment closely to the ability to pay' (Baggott 2004: 131). This is a source of concern for many commentators. Bergmark (2000) claims that those who argue in favour of private insurance schemes also tend to believe that the right to health care should be restricted to those who have made a sufficient contribution to society. This right wing view of justice, associated in particular with neo-liberal politics, fails to take into account any responsibility that society might have to provide care for the needy and is likely to lead to further injustice (see Bergmark 2000: 400, 409). Arguments in support of private health care often assume that people are free to choose between alternative health arrangements, that they are individually responsible for their own level of income and of the life chances they have. They also fail to take into account the ways in which affluent sections of society might lobby the government to reduce spending on health care. It should be recognized that those who can afford private health care are generally in a privileged position (Loewy 1999: 314–16). Moreover, reliance upon private health care not only ignores the presence of social inequalities but can also add to these inequalities. Iain Gilmour (1992), a Conservative minister who fell out of favour with the Thatcher regime, pointed out that there are limits to what the private sector can provide because vast sections of the population are unable to afford health insurance premiums and because we are most likely to need health care when we are least able to afford it. Because of this, those who are critical of the continued existence of social inequalities view private health care with some suspicion. Arguments like this will only tend to have an impact upon those who are critical of social inequalities. People who believe that inequality is both natural and unavoidable are less likely to be concerned about the impact of private practice upon levels of inequality in society.

The perils of self-interest

Critics of private health care have pointed out that the pursuit of profit and the dominance of self-interest can be socially harmful. The pursuit of profits by the private sector could be seen as creating significant barriers to appropriate care of patients. It has been argued, for example, that the profit motive creates incentives to over-provide by offering unnecessary levels of treatment so as to charge patients more (Baggott 2004). Charles Kennedy (2001) believes that the profit motive stands in the way of the private sector satisfying the health needs of the nation. For some critics, patients suffer when health care providers are motivated by commercial concerns. Loewy (1999) argues that under a system of private health care there can be conflict in the obligations felt by medics because they are often expected to serve the interests of their organizations (and their shareholders) rather than the interests of patients. The moral consequences of this can be far-reaching. According to Julian Le Grand, key figures in the public sector are more likely to be motivated by altruism, while economic motives are far more common among the managers of the private sector. He believes, moreover, that it is morally superior to work for the betterment of others than to be motivated by self-interest (Le Grand 2001: 5–6). What stimulates health care providers is thus considered of fundamental importance by critics of private health care and by some health professionals (see Box 3.2) but is largely ignored by supporters of private health care.

Box 3.2   Health professionals' critiques of private health care

Health professionals have claimed that the profit motive has a detrimental effect upon patient care. Edward Harris, a retired physician, criticized the private sector because financial incentives might prevent doctors from referring patients to others for a second opinion and this might lead doctors to take on things for which they lack the necessary qualifications and experience (Harris 1999: 96). It is argued that the profit motive pushes physicians to make decisions based upon economic criteria rather than upon patient needs. Key figures in the Registered Nurses of Ontario have argued that the public health system in Canada will often be left to finance expensive procedures while physicians take on simpler and more profitable treatment in their private practice (CBC News 2007). Health professionals have also argued that private practice is not suited to many areas of health and social care. Occupational therapists, for example, have pointed out that the state system is crucial in the field of occupational therapy because those who are in need of support are often unable to pay for private treatment (Brandis 2000). It is not simply a matter of whether an individual can afford a particular procedure but to what extent the profit motive has a negative effect upon the care we receive. We would not gain much insight into the attitudes of people towards the private sector simply by asking whether they would be willing or able to pay for a hip replacement, tattoo removal or drugs for smoking-related illnesses. Selecting a condition and asking people to imagine they had a need to access a certain type of care would only provide us with information about attitudes towards certain conditions and not necessarily tell us a great deal about attitudes towards private practice and towards the profit motive.

According to critics of private health, those involved in the design and administration of private health care plans have a vested interest in limiting or withholding health care from those they insure. Health insurance schemes are often included as part of an employment package and it is suggested that many employers are interested in spending as little as possible and so might leave their employees with inadequate cover (Loewy 1999: 318). The cover provided by managed health care plans in the United States, which allows for groups of physicians to enter into a contract with insurance groups to provide a block of services for clients of the insurance group, has been criticized by Churchill (1999: 397–408) for the following reasons:

- Managed care groups might be too preoccupied with cutting costs and physicians might find that they are offered financial incentives to cut costs. Such measures rarely benefit the patient and are more likely to advance the interests of health care professionals and insurance companies.
- Large commercial organizations can have a harmful effect upon the health care system. Profit motives and commercial interests can sit uneasily alongside the professional ethics of medics.
- Managed care is likely to exclude the 'economically unattractive'. This group, which probably includes the elderly, the poor and people suffering from AIDS, will often be forced to rely upon the limited provision offered by the state.
- Churchill believes that access to health care should be given to all sections of society regardless of their risk-rating or the amount they

are likely to consume in medical resources. Only in this way can we avoid discriminating against vulnerable sections of society.

These arguments provide another illustration of how the need to make profits can stand in the way of people gaining adequate or suitable health care.

The need for confidentiality

How important is confidentiality in health care? Should our medical records be available to a third party? Woodward (2001) argues that insurers and employers who buy health insurance packages for their workers want an increasing amount of information about the people they insure and that this threatens the autonomy of patients and their rights to confidential medical treatment. Patients are effectively tracked through their lives and evaluated on economic/risk grounds by insurers and employers alike. It is increasingly the case, especially in the United States, that the relationships between medical professionals and their patients are embedded in what has become known as the 'health care industry' (Woodward 2001: 337–40). It is questionable whether the private sector should be allowed to have access to this kind of information. Under a system of private health care which makes extensive use of insurance packages (rather than the individual paying a fee for each service received), employers and insurance companies seem to have assumed the power to monitor their employees and clients respectively. Apart from anything else, this is incompatible with the rights of patients to confidential health care.

The problem of regulation

The private sector has also been criticized for the way that it has traditionally evaded regulation. There has been some concern about standards in private health care. After the death of her husband following an unsuccessful operation in a private hospital, Emma Nicholson (a liberal peer and Euro MP) began to investigate standards in private health care and found that private hospitals often eluded regulation and that standards could therefore not be guaranteed (Sampson 2000). Private practice in Britain was often free from many of the regulations imposed upon the public sector. The Labour government, to tighten regulatory procedures, introduced the Care Standards Bill of 2000. This Bill allowed for a greater level of inspection of private health care providers and for the closure of health care facilities if they were deemed to be unsatisfactory. The Labour government declared that it is committed to monitoring and enforcing standards of care across the wide spectrum of health care providers (DH 1999; Hansard 2000). In the United States, there are considerable concerns over quality of care because the federal government seems to lack the power to enforce standards on those who provide private health care (Dranove 2000). In the European Union, private health insurers have been given greater freedom to offer health insurance across the European Union.

This has reduced the ability of individual governments to regulate the private health care market in their own countries (Thomson and Mossialos 2004: 2). While private health care providers resist regulation, we might wish to treat with scepticism the assertion that private practitioners provide a superior service to the state. This is, of course, a controversial issue. If we choose to access private health care, should this be seen as a commercial transaction between us and the state? Can comparisons be made with buying any other product or service? We can shop around, compare prices and make decisions about what we want and what we can afford. If the state is involved in regulating the private sector, does this give the state too many powers over the economic transactions between patients and private health care providers? From a neo-liberal point of view, the answer to this question is probably yes. Those who are more supportive of state involvement, however, may wish to point out that the state is often needed to protect citizens from the unscrupulous activities of private businesses.

Scenario 7   Illustration of the potential disadvantages of the private sector

Let us think once again about Edna, the 85-year-old woman who is housebound after a recent operation. She has health insurance but can only afford limited cover and therefore can only receive assistance three times a week. She has little support in deciding which might be the best health care provider and has therefore chosen the one she has seen in television adverts. This happens to be the most expensive. Edna is not happy with the quality of care she receives but has no family to help her and does not know where to turn for support.

Questions

You are a health care worker attached to a local primary care provider. You become aware of Edna's circumstances.

1   What, if anything, could you do to assist Edna?
2   To what extent should health care workers in the state sector help patients access suitable services from the private sector?

The resolution of differences

It might be that the distinction between the state provision of health care versus heavy reliance upon private health care is out of tune with the character of our times and that we should look to devise an affordable and fair combination of public and private provision. The state would be there to care for all who needed it alongside a vibrant system of private health care for those who can afford it (see Ashcroft et al. 2000: 390). For the Blair government in Britain, it was important to find ways for the NHS to make use of the private sector. Hutton (2004) argued that the NHS is in need of fundamental reform. The original aims of the service were no longer seen as suitable or credible for increasingly affluent citizens with heightened expectations. In Hutton's view, the NHS must be able to accommodate different expectations, extend choice to patients and as part of this process renegotiate relations between the public and private sectors. In particular, Hutton argued that the NHS should make greater use of both private sector managerial skills and of private sector facilities so as to extend the range of services available to patients. It is clear that for some the private sector is seen as an important provider of health care even under the umbrella of a largely nationalized state health service. Questions remain over how these services are to be paid for, but at least if the government enters into negotiations with the private sector it seems likely that the state health system will be transformed. This of course might mean that the public sector is streamlined and the private sector expands in certain areas. Viewed cynically, such a move might be necessary to allow governments to manage and tame our expectations of the NHS. The view that we should think increasingly in terms of a mixed economy of health care does have some support from health care professionals (see Box 3.3).

Box 3.3   Health professionals and the mixed economy of health

Health professionals have become increasingly willing to embrace the advantages of a mixed economy of care. For example, the British Medical Association (BMA) concluded in 2001 that a state funded health care system was preferable to private health care but that private health care must still have a place for those procedures not covered by the NHS. The BMA stated that the NHS should no longer see itself as providing a comprehensive service and that it is necessary to acknowledge that rationing and denial of service also exists in state health care (Morris 2001). Support for a mixed economy of care often stems from a pragmatic understanding that a comprehensive state health service is difficult to sustain. Factors including increased life expectancy and the use of expensive technology have placed a strain on state-funded health care systems and forced many governments to look for ways to protect core services by placing limits upon what is funded by the state. Governments have attempted to reduce expenditure on health care by diverting resources into health promotion (see Chapter 6), using rationing techniques (see Chapter 7) or through leaving some areas of health care to private practice or to voluntary groups (see Chapter 4).

If the boundaries between the public and private sectors can be renegotiated, this will no doubt have to involve a shift in the moral value we ascribe to both sectors. Public service and private profit seem at first glance to have little in common, but those looking to redesign relations between the public and private sectors try to look beyond the motives of different providers and give greater credence to the outcomes of their actions. Julian Le Grand, for example, believes that governments and policy makers might have to trade off the moral advantages of public provision against the 'equally valid moral claims relating to outcomes' (Le Grand 2001: 15). Le Grand argues that altruistic acts are not necessarily better for the welfare of others and that it is necessary to judge the impact of an action not merely the motivation behind an act. Although he acknowledges that altruism is more prevalent among public sector managers, he rejects the view that those in the public sector are the only ones spurred on by such motives. He claims that although it is morally desirable for people to be motivated by altruism rather than by self-interest, it must surely be desirable that health care is also improved. Given that private companies can provide high quality health care, he argues that it makes sense for us to use these companies 'regardless of the impact this has on the stock of altruism in society' (Le Grand 2001: 14). In short, we need to consider to what extent the motives of those who provide health care are of any importance. If, like Le Grand, we focus instead upon maximizing the numbers who receive treatment then our resistance to private health care may well start to crumble. Does it matter who provides health care as long as patient needs are tended to? If the answer is no, there is plenty of scope for the private sector to offer a range of services.

Scenario 8   Illustration of a mixed approach to health care

Let us return to consider Edna, the 85-year-old woman who is housebound after a recent hip operation. If you recall, she has some health care provision through the state but also chooses to 'top up' her care by paying for someone to come into her home and provide her with additional support.

Questions

1   To what extent do you think that mixed provision of care can work well and tend to the needs of the patient?
2   What do you think are the benefits and disadvantages of this approach?
3   To what extent can this approach provide a suitable alternative to relying solely upon the state or private provision?
4   Are there any disadvantages to mixed provision of care?

Policy developments

When we talk about approaches to private health care, we need to bear in mind that the most effective way to promote private health care is to reduce the resources available for state health care. If the state refuses or is unable to provide certain types of treatment or accommodate the vast numbers seeking care, then it effectively forces people to look for alternatives. State health care tends to be seen as essential for emergency cover and for acute illnesses, but rather less so for chronic conditions (arthritis, asthma, diabetes and so on) and for what could be regarded as repair work (for example, hip replacements or restorative surgery). It would appear that people will often turn towards private health care when their conditions are assigned a low priority in state health care systems. Private practitioners seem particularly good at offering to reduce suffering (for a price) rather than having to deal with medical emergencies.

Britain

The desirability or otherwise of private health care has been a hot political issue in Britain. The two main political parties in Britain (the Conservative Party and the Labour Party) owe their origins to radically different views of the world and attempt to make their primary appeal to different social classes. Traditionally, the Labour Party has relied upon the support of the working class and, as we will see, has pointed out on numerous occasions that the working class cannot generally afford private health care, private education and even private ownership of housing. The traditional audience and supporters of the Conservative Party tend to be more prosperous and are generally more able to afford to tend to their own health, education and housing needs. This class division, reflected in the ideas and policies of the two main political parties, is far from absolute and is subject to change over time. The Conservative and Labour parties can no longer rely solely upon the support of the relatively prosperous and the relatively poor respectively. Political parties have found increasingly that they are struggling to gain the attention and support of a huge middle ground of people on modest incomes with little or no interest in politics (see Todd and Taylor 2004). The swelling of this so-called 'Middle England' has in turn had an impact upon the views expressed by the main political parties.

The Conservative Party

Private health care has received sustained support from the Conservative Party in Britain. The Conservative Party has often argued in favour of maintaining elements of private practice within the NHS (Conservative Party 1955). Whereas the Labour Party frequently saw the private sector as a threat to the state health system, the Conservatives believed that people need to be free to make choices about the health care they receive and the freedom to provide for their own families if they so wish (Conservative Party 1970a). The Conservative Party (1970b) argued that the abolition of private practice within the NHS was unacceptable because it would deprive the NHS of funds and would reduce the health care available to patients. Up until the mid-1970s, the Conservative Party supported the private sector on fairly pragmatic grounds. Although it took some time for the Conservatives to accept the NHS, for much of the immediate post-war period Conservatives seemed content to argue that private practice should be allowed to develop alongside state provision.

The tone of Conservative arguments changed considerably during the late 1970s. The rise of Margaret Thatcher and the spread of neo-liberal ideas helped to project the private sector as a worthy competitor and possible successor to state health care. In 1979, the Conservative Party made it clear that it was in favour of a radical review of the NHS and that this review would consider the possible role of health insurance as a source for funding state health care (Conservative Party 1979). The Conservative Party (1983) argued that the Labour Party was wrong to expect the state to do everything and that a lot could be gained from developing partnerships with the private sector. Private practice was seen as particularly important for covering non-urgent operations and as such provided a valuable supplement to the state provision of health care. The Thatcher governments gave tax subsidies to individuals and employers as a way to encourage them to use private health care. These governments promoted the view that private health care provided a better and morally superior service to that being offered by the NHS. The Conservatives claimed that the private sector was far more efficient and responsive to consumer needs and that the public sector was inherently flawed because it was shielded from the pressure of competition. It has been suggested that the Thatcher governments were responsible for 'the expansion of the commercial sector ideal to the point of undermining the solidaristic foundations of the welfare state itself' (Ackers and Abbott 1996: 116). The private sector, not only in health care but also in other areas of economic and social life, was viewed by the Thatcher governments in an extremely positive light and as having the potential to lead Britain out of economic decline and its apparent dependency upon the welfare state. The desire for profit was considered fundamental to human nature and an essential motivating force that could help in Britain's economic and social renaissance.

There were limits, however, to what the Conservatives were willing to do. During the late 1980s, the Conservatives considered privatizing vast areas of health care and of using tax breaks to secure support. This was considered to be politically unattractive and was thus dropped from the policy agenda (BBC2 1996a). Rather than look for ways to privatize health care, the Conservatives have been more prone to promote the virtues of the private sector while recognizing the necessity of maintaining the NHS. In 1995, the Conservative government rejected calls by Healthcare 2000 (a project funded privately by drug companies) to limit the public provision of health care to core services only and to rely increasingly on the extension of private health care (Suzman, 1995; Brindle, 1995). The Conservatives floated the idea in 2003 of giving patients the option to receive partial funding for private treatment as a way to reduce the pressure on waiting lists and mounting health expenditure. The Conservative Party insisted that this would in no way threaten the right of people to receive free treatment but that it did at least provide a way to help rather than to penalize those who wish to access private health care (Beattie 2003). For the Conservatives, it has become more important to recognize the contribution that can be made by private health to the mixed economy of health care. Although it would seem that the Conservatives have a soft spot for the private sector, this is not strong enough to urge them to challenge the apparent widespread support for state health care in Britain.

The Labour Party

The Labour Party has traditionally been quite critical of private health care. Social democrats in general are hostile towards the private sector, largely because it allows for people to be exploited and because it operates more often than not to maximize profits. For social democrats (and social democratic parties like the Labour Party) the economic and social systems need to be ordered to ensure that all citizens have opportunities for work and access to decent housing, education and health care (see Taylor 2007). As we saw in the previous chapter, when the Labour government created the NHS in 1948 it allowed for the continuation of private practice inside the NHS and it left some hospitals in private hands. Although this was deemed necessary to ensure the compliance of the powerful consultants, it was to remain a source of embarrassment for Labour administrations into the 1970s. The National Union of Public Employees and the Labour Minister Barbara Castle led a campaign to remove private practice from inside the NHS. Although the Labour government reduced the amount of private practice in the NHS, this was seen as little more than a gesture (see Ackers and Abbott 1996; BBC2 1995). Out of office between 1979 and 1997, the Labour Party continued to be critical of the private sector in health care. In 1983, the Labour Party pledged to end private practice in the NHS and called for the end of all public subsidies to the private sector. It was argued that the existence of private practice within the NHS creates a two-tier health service in which those with money could jump the queue for treatment (Labour Party 1983). In the run up to both the 1987 and the 1992 General Elections, the Labour Party reaffirmed its opposition to the private sector. By then, it was worried that the Conservative Party was effectively privatizing the health service to the detriment of patients' needs and interests (Labour Party 1987; Labour Party 1992). In particular, the Labour Party criticized the Conservatives for attempting to create a service that could be run along business lines (Labour Party 1992). Traditional Labour Party philosophy is embedded firmly in social democratic ideas and gives far more credence to our social rights than to what is business-like. The Labour Party was for many years willing to finance a large public sector in the belief that this would benefit British citizens in a variety of ways. The priority was social justice, almost regardless of cost.

New Labour and the third way
When the Labour Party returned to office in 1997, it was a different beast driven by different ideas. Tired from its prolonged period in opposition, it transformed its theoretical base and started to talk about a third way in which the public and private sectors could exist alongside each other and cooperate in a multitude of economic and social ventures. The Labour Party's attitude towards the private sector was transformed. Faced with an NHS in serious need of investment, the Labour Party embraced with minimal embarrassment the so-called Private Finance Initiative. According to the Labour government in Britain, the Private Finance Initiative provided an opportunity to establish an effective partnership between the public and private sectors in which the private sector risked its own money in the production of high quality public services. The government was keen to point out that the private sector would have to bear the costs if any project ran over budget (HM Treasury 2006; HM Treasury 2007). Tony Blair claimed in his keynote address to the Confederation of British Industry's Public Services Summit in January 2007 that the private sector has always been involved in construction projects in the health service and that what the Private Finance Initiative offers is a way to ensure that these projects are completed within an agreed budget and on time (PPP Forum 2007). The Labour government was thus willing to increase the functions of the private sector in the NHS.

Labour's sudden change of heart has been justified in a number of ways. Paul Boateng, the financial secretary to the British Treasury, placed the Private Finance Initiative into a broader policy framework. He claimed that it was essential to reform and modernize the public services and that this was the dominant policy agenda for the Labour government's second term of office (which ran from 2001–2005). Boateng claimed that the Blair government had a pragmatic rather than an ideological approach to investment in the public sector. Rather than praise the public sector and condemn the private sector, Boateng suggested that each case should be evaluated according to its outputs. If the private sector helped to deliver public facilities and services at a high standard, then it deserved support (Hansard 2001). Senior members of the Labour Party believed that it was time to put aside ideological objections to the private sector and Tony Blair was open about his commitment to break down the barriers between the private, voluntary and public sectors. In his view, this issue went beyond ideology and he believed that the aspiration to remove these barriers had widespread support (PPP Forum 2007). For Gordon Brown, the Private Finance Initiative was in the public interest and he believed that it provided a way for the government to enter into partnerships with the private sector and to use its innovative techniques and strong managerial skills to deliver high quality public facilities (PPP Forum 2007). For New Labour, the private sector can have a significant role in regenerating the public sector and advancing the public interest.

The weakness of opposition parties

It does of course help that there is no real opposition from the Conservative Party or from the Liberal Democrats to making use of the private sector in health care. According to the Conservative Party (1997), partnerships with the private sector could be used to enhance capital investment in the NHS. The Conservative Party therefore pledged its support to the Private Finance Initiative in the belief that this could be used to provide the funds necessary to modernize the foundations of the state health system. The Conservative Party, which took credit for introducing the Private Finance Initiative, claim that it has become important for the Labour government because it has provided the government with a way to conceal its expenditure on public services (Hansard 2002). The Liberal Democrat Party, while not overtly critical of the private sector, is rather less impressed by the ability of the Private Finance Initiative to deliver real value for money and favours instead the use of private sector management rather than private sector finance. According to the Liberal Democrat Party, herein lies the real strength of the private sector (Hansard 2001). As we have noted, the private sector now has widespread support across the main political parties in Britain. It is seen as having the potential to mobilize some of the new resources needed to modernize the NHS. It has not, however, always gained support from health professionals (see Box 3.4).

Box 3.4   Health professionals and the Private Finance Initiative

The Private Finance Initiative is likely to have a dramatic impact upon the health service in Britain and to those who work within the state sector. It provides an opportunity to modernize facilities but at a price. Some members of the health professions have viewed the Private Finance Initiative with suspicion, especially in its early years. In 1996, the British Medical Association criticized the Private Finance Initiative in the belief that this initiative will be used to privatize the NHS. It was argued that the Conservative government was failing to acknowledge the realities of under-funding in the NHS and that it was coercing hospitals to use private funding. The Private Finance Initiative was described as 'covert privatisation' (Anon 1996). Health service managers have also been critical of the Private Finance Initiative because it led in its early stages to severe cuts in capital expenditure in the NHS and because it created unnecessary layers of bureaucracy and delay (see Suzman 1997).

United States

It has been acknowledged that health care in the United States is delivered by a multitude of agencies that have no real connections with each other. It is said that the federal government is not in the business of creating a uniform health system but of working alongside private businesses to maintain quality in care, fairness in price and reliable information on health and health care (US Department of Health and Human Services 2007b). Governments have sought to encourage people in the United States to use private health care by providing tax breaks to those who take out private health insurance. President George W. Bush offered tax relief to people who buy their own health care packages and has argued that federal government should avoid playing a major role in the provision of health care and that citizens should be able to make decisions about the level of health care they want and are willing to pay for (Bush 2004). Private health care is extremely important in the United States and is often seen as preferable to federal or state health care provision.

The Republican Party

Like the Conservative Party in Britain, the Republican Party in the United States is a staunch defender of private health care. The Republican Party argues that individuals get a better service through participation in private health insurance schemes and that attempts should be made to extend the number of people covered by private policies through giving tax relief to those paying private premiums. It is recognized, however, that some citizens are unable to afford private cover and that for these people the federal government should fund some basic health care (Republican Party 2007). For the Republican Party, using tax breaks to encourage more people to take out private health cover is thought to empower individuals and to allow us to take more control and indeed ownership over our own health and health care. According to this view, citizens need to rely less upon the 'nanny state', be willing to assume more responsibility for their health and exercise more choice over the health care they buy (American Presidency Project 2007b). It is clear that George W. Bush is against excessive federal involvement in health care. Instead, he believes that the private sector should be valued because it gives more choice to the consumer and because it nourishes relations between doctors and patients. He believes that it could also be good in labour relations, as many employers provide health insurance cover for their employees (American Presidency Project

2004). For the Republicans, our freedom depends upon us having control over our own money and upon making decisions about our own lives. From a Republican perspective, government intervention in the economic and social systems is regarded as intrusive and a threat to the freedom of the individual. It therefore makes perfect sense for the Republicans to promote the virtues of the private sector and to support private health care.

The Democratic Party

The Democratic Party is considerably less confident in the ability of the private sector to cater for the health needs of the American nation. The Democrats have pointed out that insurance companies, drug companies and the lobbyists who represent these interests have done everything they can to prevent the American government from making a commitment to providing universal health care (American Presidency Project 2007b). Democrats have argued that the system of private health insurance stands in the way of real care because insurance companies make a profit from denying care. Because of this, it is argued that Medicare (currently available for the elderly) should be extended to all people and in so doing help to undermine the influence of private insurance companies (American Presidency Project 2007b). President Obama declared his support for the expansion of health insurance to a greater number of American citizens. Included among his proposals was the development of a new system of tax credits for small businesses to assist them in providing health insurance for their workers. Small businesses were also encouraged to consider a range of options available with the help of a National Health Insurance Exchange, in which private providers outlined what they had to offer (Obama and Biden 2009). The Democratic Party is far closer to the ideological complexion of New Labour. The private sector is viewed as useful but not suitable as the sole provider of health care in the United States. It is apparent that the Democrats are more concerned than the Republicans with the welfare of those who are unable to afford suitable health care. This stems from two different world views. For the Republicans, self-help is applauded and valued above government aid. For the Democrats, we must be willing to look out for each other and be willing to use government programmes to advance the common welfare.

International comparisons

The private sector tends to be vibrant where individuals are largely responsible for their own health care. The private sector in the United States falls into this category. Where health care is financed through taxation, the state will tend to have a greater role in the provision of health care. This would apply to Britain, Canada, Australia, New Zealand and to countries in Scandinavia. Health systems based upon social insurance are more likely to have a mix between public and private provision. This would apply to France, Germany and to the Netherlands (see Stewart 1999). The difference between these health systems is, however, far from extreme. Since the late 1990s even those systems that rely heavily upon active state involvement in the provision of health care have turned increasingly towards the private sector. As we saw when discussing recent developments in Britain, many governments have come to believe that a large state health service is unsustainable and hopes to convince at least some people to use private health care.

Canada, Australia and New Zealand

Canada, Australia and New Zealand allow for a mix between public and private provision. Recent developments in Canada have allowed more room for the private sector. The provinces in Canada have always varied in their support of state health care. While Quebec has tended to favour government intervention, such intervention has tended to be viewed with suspicion by provincial governments in Alberta. Health spending has, however, been cut in a variety of provinces including Quebec, Alberta and Ontario. The more this occurs, the more people have to rely upon the private sector (see Crichton et al. 1997). Governments in Australia and New Zealand likewise gave more scope to the private sector during the 1990s. The number of private beds in hospitals doubled in New Zealand between 1958 and the early 1990s. Governments, in the hope of relieving pressure on the state health system, have actively encouraged this (Flood 2000). The Australian Government has also attempted to revive private health care. Between 1985 and 1999, there was a rapid decline in the number of Australian people holding private medical insurance. Convinced that the Australian Medicare system was in danger of collapse, the Australian government argued that a well-funded private sector was essential to relieve the pressure on the state health care system. The Australian government therefore introduced generous rebates on insurance premiums in the hope of convincing more people to make use of private health care (see Vaithianathan 2002). Policy makers have been driven by the need to maintain equity of access to public health care while promoting the expansion of the private sector in the interests of increasing efficiency and patient choice (Colombo and Tapay 2003: 4). Canada, New Zealand and Australia could be seen as reluctant advocates of private health care. They have recognized, along with Britain, that encouraging those who can afford to access private health care might be necessary to save health care provided by the state.

Sweden

The pressure to privatize has hit some of the staunchest supporters of state health care. Although Sweden has a long tradition of extensive public provision of health care, there was a marked increase in private practitioners in primary care during the 1980s and 1990s (Whitehead et al. 1997). During the 1980s, popular support for the welfare state in Sweden fell and people became increasingly critical of bureaucratic procedures and mistrustful of those entitled to benefits. As people became more confident about their own economic prospects, they began to believe that they would have little need for the welfare state in their own futures and thus tended to support measures to privatize sections of the welfare state. Economic decline during the 1990s, however, turned many people against excessive privatization and made them reassess the value of the welfare state. As a result of these changing conditions, people became more willing to pay higher taxes to fund welfare services (Bergmark 2000: 406–7). It would appear, indeed, that private provision might be attractive during periods of economic prosperity but that it becomes less popular during times of slump in the economy. It would seem that lacking money and/or security in one's own work can increase the appeal of the public sector and make us view the private sector as offering something beyond our reach.

Conclusion

Depending upon your political views, the private sector can be seen as anything ranging from ultra-modern providers of high quality service to pariahs seeking to profit from human suffering. Supporters of private health care emphasize the responsibilities we have for our own health and health care and point out that state health care systems serve as an unnecessary drain upon national resources partly because there is no real limit to what people will demand from the public sector. Under private health care, patients tend to be far more restrained in what they seek to access. This market discipline appeals in particular to neo-liberals and is seen in the party programmes of the Conservative Party in Britain and the Republican Party in the United States. Health professionals might find this attractive because of the emphasis placed upon innovative practice and because of the attention paid to providing high quality facilities. However, critics of private health care doubt whether patients receive adequate care because such care cuts into the profits of private health care providers. For the critics, people have an equal right to health care regardless of their ability to pay. These critics include the Labour Party in Britain and the Democratic Party in the United States. Working under a state health care system, the virtues of altruism are likely to be given greater value than those of profit. Despite this chasm between health care for profit and health care as a public service, state health care systems have been under significant strain. This has prompted many advocates of state health care to find ways to encourage the development of the private sector in the hope of relieving some of the pressure upon state health care. As we have seen, this applies in particular to the British Labour Party since 1997 and to the development of health care in Australia, Canada, New Zealand and Sweden. It is becoming recognized increasingly that state health care might not be able to satisfy all of our health needs and that the private sector might be necessary to extend choice and convenience to those who can afford private treatment. The message appears to be clear. State health care is in trouble, especially if we discard the contribution that can be made by private practice.

4   The voluntary sector

Chapter Contents

So far, the choice seems quite clear. Either we rely upon the state to provide us with health care or we pay for our own. Those who want the state to assume responsibility often do so in the belief that we have social rights to health care. For those who support the private sector, it is more important that we recognize our responsibilities for ourselves. But the choice is not restricted to these polar positions. The voluntary sector, a term that is often used to refer to charities and to groups that exist in the community, provides policy makers with another alternative means to deliver health care. It also raises a number of other questions about our responsibilities towards each other, for example:

- What would you be prepared to give freely to strangers?
- Why should you give anything, especially if you live in a country with a well-funded welfare state?
- If you pay taxes, is that enough or do your social and moral obligations toward the community extend beyond this?

People who are deciding whether or not to engage in voluntary activity might ask themselves such questions. We could argue that we are all members of the community and what happens in that community will eventually impact upon us all. Could engaging in voluntary activity provide us with an indirect way to maintain our own long-term interests? The voluntary sector provides a means by which people can, if they wish, make a contribution to society and to the communities in which they live.

The voluntary sector compared with other sectors

The voluntary sector is the third main provider of health care covered in this volume. Whereas the state often intervenes to promote the public good and the private sector is more often than not motivated by the desire for profit, voluntary sector groups often work in local communities and are constituted to represent the needs of specific groups of people. Perhaps the distinction between these various sectors can be seen in the following way. In order to access health care facilities owned and controlled by the state you need to be recognized as a citizen of that particular country. If you are a British citizen, for example, you are entitled to health care through the NHS. Alternatively, you might have rights to health care stemming from arrangements made between your government and the government in control of the health care you want to access. British citizens, for example, can access some health care facilities in other European states as a result of arrangements made between the British government and other member states of the European Union. To secure private health care, you need to be able to afford to pay the fee or be covered by an insurance package recognized by the particular private health care provider. To make use of voluntary sector services, you need first to be able to find suitable voluntary sector groups. General practitioners and hospitals can often help by providing links or referrals and might be willing to do so not only for the benefit of the patient but also to relieve the pressure on their services. Patients, however, need not fear that this will cost them a great deal. The services provided by voluntary sector groups are often free or heavily subsidized by the state or as a condition of the funding they receive. Voluntary sector groups can therefore make a vast difference to those who are looking for an alternate or supplement to state health care or to those who are unable to visit private practitioners.

The character and functions of the voluntary sector

When the term voluntary sector is used it may well conjure up images of charity shops and collection boxes. This is a rather narrow image of the voluntary sector and one we stray from in the current chapter. Although the voluntary sector often makes use of volunteers, many groups in the voluntary sector employ workers to manage projects and to apply for funding. The voluntary sector is indeed now one of the largest employers in Britain. It is formally separate from the state, relatively autonomous, self-governing and involved in service delivery on a non-profit making basis. The survival of voluntary sector groups, however, relies to a large extent upon government support. Although voluntary sector groups might raise some of the money they need from public donations or from fund-raising events, they often find that their survival is dependent upon securing grants from the statutory sector. These grants are necessary to pay their workers and to finance voluntary sector projects and activities (see Todd and Ware 2001).

Voluntary sector groups perform a number of roles. These have been categorized by Todd and Ware (2001) in the following way:

- *Service providers*: for example, the Citizens Advice Bureau;
- *Mutual aid and self-help groups*: these are often based on identity (age, gender, sexuality, ethnicity, etc.);
- *Campaigning groups*: for example, the Child Poverty Action Group;
- *Advocacy groups*: for example, MIND;
- *Coordinating groups*: for example, the National Council for Voluntary Organizations;
- *Leisure Groups*: these offer a range of activities including education, dance, music and so on.

The list above is by no means exhaustive but it has been included to illustrate some of the diversity within the voluntary sector. It is clear, however, that while some groups could be regarded as providing front-line services for a client group, others work behind the scenes to campaign for changes in the law, raise awareness or coordinate smaller groups. The voluntary sector, indeed, should be seen as a network of inter-related groups that have relations with each other and with the statutory and private sectors.

Political perspectives on the voluntary sector

The voluntary sector is seen in a positive light by many of the mainstream political ideologies. Although generally in favour of state activity, social democrats recognize that the voluntary sector can be viewed as a vehicle of compassion towards each other and a sign of what can be achieved through collective effort (see Peckham and Meerabeau 2007; Taylor 2007). For neo-liberals, the voluntary sector should be at the heart of welfare provision and is preferred over using the state. Milton Friedman, for example, argued that state intervention in economic and social life often failed to have the desired effect because it attempted to subordinate individual interests to the general good. In so doing, he believed that state intervention also threatened our wish to contribute to our communities freely through voluntary activity (see Friedman 1962; Ackers and Abbott 1996). For proponents of the third way, the voluntary sector opens up possibilities for transforming the role of the state from the provider to the coordinator of many public services and for attracting people to participate in social and political life. Anthony Giddens (2000) believes that if developed effectively the voluntary sector can help to mature our civic culture, assist in the regeneration of communities and 'can offer choice and responsiveness in the delivery of public services' (Giddens 2000: 81; see also Wilding 2002; Peckham and Meerabeau 2007). The widespread appeal of the voluntary sector has allowed governments of various political persuasions to delegate some of their functions to voluntary groups. As we shall see, it has become particularly important in the context of the state reducing its role in health care.

Theoretical perspectives

When attempting to construct a theoretical framework that can be used in discussions on the voluntary sector, we have placed special emphasis upon identifying the strengths of the voluntary sector and contrasting these with the problems it faces. Whereas our coverage of theoretical perspectives on the state and the private sector looked at the arguments for and against each of these, it was decided that there was considerably more mileage in attempting to look at the voluntary sector according to the problems it faces and what it needs to develop rather than to ask whether or not it should exist. We have seen that the state is in the process of withdrawing from intervening in many areas of economic and social life and we should bear in mind that if the state continues to withdraw from social provision its place has to be taken by some other sector. As we have seen, the private sector alone cannot guarantee the public good. The voluntary sector therefore provides an alternative source of provision for those who recognize the social context of health and health care and our broader social responsibilities.

The strengths of the voluntary sector

One of the key strengths of the voluntary sector lies in its workforce. It is often noted how workers in the voluntary sector tend to be committed to their communities or areas of interest and are thus motivated to innovate and contribute towards the development of their organization. The voluntary sector provides opportunities for people who are interested in the welfare of a particular section of the community. For example, there could be opportunities to work with children, people from ethnic minority backgrounds or with people who define their identity in terms of a particular sexuality. People who work in the voluntary sector often have to be innovative in the way they contact, communicate and intervene in the community. The Liberal/SDP Alliance (1987) claimed that the voluntary sector is important in health care, partly because of the enthusiastic workers it attracts and the diverse methods it employs. It is recognized that the skills developed in the voluntary sector are of considerable value and that the statutory sector has much it can learn from these non-state groups (see DH 1998b; DH 2004a: 79). When committed and focussed, the voluntary sector can shine brightly and provide an excellent service.

Information and communication

Voluntary groups tend to work in local communities and can therefore provide important information and expertise for policy makers at local, national and international levels. The information gathered and research conducted by voluntary sector groups can often have a beneficial impact upon policy deliberations. The British government in particular has been interested in attracting contributions towards policy debates from voluntary groups (DH 2001d: 18). The World Health Organisation likewise values the information and insights of the voluntary sector and believes the voluntary sector can make interesting contributions to the policy making process. It is suggested that voluntary groups often work effectively to communicate need and to exert pressure for improvements in services. This role is particularly important in the field of mental heath (WHO 2003: 7; WHO 2004: 25). What makes the voluntary sector so important is that it can provide different types of information and insight into problems. It can identify the needs of its client groups and point to gaps in existing provision. In addition to declaring what needs to be done, voluntary groups are well placed to identify how policies should be formulated and implemented. Such links with the community make voluntary sector groups experts on the specific needs and dispositions of their client groups.

The comfort of the familiar

The voluntary sector can seem less daunting to clients than services provided by the state. By making use of voluntary groups in the delivery of services, barriers to the effective implementation of policies can be reduced. According to the World Health Organisation (2003), mental health services provided by the voluntary sector in the community are important because they provide the first point of contact for those who do not wish or are unable to access services provided by the state. What is provided by the voluntary sector is often readily available and tends to be accepted by clients because voluntary groups are located in familiar surroundings. A lot of this is down to the way we perceive the state and whether we are confident that the state can provide us with suitable treatment. Somehow, and this might be heartfelt by people in a vulnerable condition, what is on offer in the local community might seem less alienating than the services offered by the state or the private sector.

Cultural sensitivity

The voluntary sector seems particularly well suited to adapt to the needs of different groups of people and to inform the state and other funding bodies of those needs. It is recognized that the statutory sector is unable to gauge the health needs of the community in general and of marginalized sections of the community in particular (see, for example, NIMHE 2003: 23). For example, western ideas of trauma and stress focus upon individual psychology. This approach is inappropriate for the treatment of non-western patients suffering from post-traumatic stress. For many non-western asylum seekers, often fleeing from tyranny and the ravages of civil war, trauma and stress are seen in the context of the community rather than solely in terms of the individual. It has been suggested that failure to understand this communal dimension could stand in the way of effective medical intervention (Silove 2004). This could be for a multitude of reasons, including the suspicion with which marginalized groups might regard the state. Involving a voluntary sector group, however, might make all the difference. Using the example outlined above, a voluntary group that included members of the particular marginalized community could act as a bridge between the asylum seekers and the state and in so doing help to provide necessary information about their health care needs. Without this information, the abilities of the state to provide appropriate services would be weakened. This would seem to apply in particular when designing services appropriate for members of ethnic minority groups (see DH 2001c: 95). In structuring appropriate services, it is important that language, culture, religion and beliefs about health are taken into account. Voluntary sector groups, often working closely with members of the community, would appear to be particularly adept at gathering and transmitting this information and thereby helping the state to understand what is needed.

Scenario 9 The role of the voluntary sector

Shamilia is a 17-year-old asylum seeker escaping persecution from her country. She is seeking asylum after her parents were arrested for their political views and tortured. She has entered the country alone and is awaiting a decision about whether she will be supported as a child or treated as an adult seeking asylum. The local asylum seeker centre is currently giving her support. Here she is given vouchers for essentials and has someone to provide translation and advocacy. She is experiencing loneliness and isolation and has therefore been enrolled on a befriending scheme provided by the centre (support is given by refugees who have been granted asylum). However, the centre's future funding has become uncertain and Shamilia is worried that she will lose the support she is being given.

Questions

You are a health care worker in the community:

1 How important is the voluntary sector in supporting Shamilia?
2 What, if anything, can be done to improve Shamilia's circumstances?

Empowering volunteers

The voluntary sector can also empower those who use and help to run the service. Webster (2002) notes how the voluntary sector is particularly good at empowering client groups to make changes to their own lifestyle and to improve their own circumstances. This empowerment takes place not only through providing information and assistance but also through encouraging groups to voice their concerns and to make links with others. He argues that this can be significant in improving the self-esteem of vulnerable people (see Webster 2002). In a fascinating account of voluntary action in the United States, Robert Wuthnow (1991) notes that over 31 million Americans volunteer every year in faith groups, 20 million volunteer in educational establishments and 16 million in health projects. His study attempts to show how voluntary action is used by many Americans to display compassion and how this often enhances their own status and standing in the community and among their peers. Using a variety of case studies, he illustrates how voluntary activity can benefit individuals emotionally, intellectually and even materially. The voluntary sector, by providing opportunities for volunteers, can have a significant impact upon the way individuals see themselves and upon a community's sense of well-being. These benefits are recognized by many health professionals (see Box 4.1).

Box 4.1 Health professionals on the strengths of the voluntary sector

Health professionals are aware of the ways in which the voluntary sector can help in the development of appropriate services. Nurses in the United States have found that working in partnership with voluntary groups like the Alzheimer's Society can help to develop a service that caters to the needs of patients and their families (Downs and Bowers 2008: 225). The voluntary sector also helps to break down some of the barriers to effective medical intervention. Nurses have found that working with and training people from the voluntary sector can often provide a useful conduit to reach 'at risk' groups in society. By working with and through volunteers in a community setting, nurses have been able to reach those who were previously suspicious of health care professionals (Kane 2008: 269). Health professionals recognize also that participating in voluntary groups can assist in recovery from illness. The British Medical Association (BMA) argues that voluntary sector involvement in health care can help members of the community see themselves as participants in the healing process and to take ownership of their own health service (BMA 2002: 29). Consultants have argued that involving people in the voluntary sector, especially in groups where clients can help each other, can often be enriching for a person's sense of self and that people who volunteer often feel better about their own health and spend less time worrying about their own health problems (Cook 2004: 10). It would seem, indeed, that the voluntary sector can help to make accessing health care less daunting for the patient through working in the patients own community and in allowing patients scope to participate in groups and put something back into their local area. It should be apparent that such opportunities are rarely provided by the state and private sectors.

Problems faced by the voluntary sector

The voluntary sector faces a number of problems. By far the most prevalent is the problem of securing sustainable sources of funding. The Liberal/SDP Alliance (1987) recognized that local authorities often exploit voluntary groups by keeping them dependent upon short-term funding and thus making them the servants of the changing priorities of government bodies. It was argued that this imbalance in power could only be remedied by securing long-term funding arrangements for voluntary groups. It has been argued that voluntary sector initiatives with ethnic minority groups are particularly unstable because of the lack of long-term funding commitments (NIMHE 2003: 23). Short-term contracts create insecurity for voluntary groups, especially if these groups are small and work with a low level of resource. This in turn can lead to problems in dedicating resources to develop new services and to recruit members of staff who are looking to establish long-term relations with a group or long-term commitment to a particular cause (Peckham and Meerabeau 2007). Those who work in the voluntary sector often do so with limited job security and find that they have to chase funding in order to secure their jobs for a little longer. Such insecurity is incompatible with the development of sustainable services. This must surely exert a negative pressure on the workers, volunteers and clients of voluntary sector groups.

Quality control and the problems of short-term funding

The voluntary sector is not necessarily constituted to ensure a consistent audit of their projects and problems can arise from using voluntary groups in service provision when these services are not audited for quality. Although public providers are subject to audit and scrutiny, mental health services in the community sometimes escape quality control (see WHO 2003: 18). This might arise, for example, when groups are evaluated according to the quantity rather than the quality of the services they provide. Commentators argue that the voluntary sector is not able to guarantee even provision and that the state is better able to guarantee access to services (Todd and Ware 2001). The ability of voluntary sector groups to be flexible in the services they offer could also be a source of weakness. The constant need to chase funding means that voluntary sector groups are constantly redesigning what they have to offer. A group representing the Chinese community, for example, might have begun by managing a social space for Chinese people but over time could find that it moves into a variety of health, education and welfare projects in an attempt to secure enough money to keep going. These groups do not always have the luxury of periods of long-term funding and stability, both of which would seem essential for the development of a specialist service.

Developing the voluntary sector

Despite these problems, it is argued that we need to look for ways to develop the voluntary sector. WHO (2004) recommend a number of measures to assist in this development including a revision of funding arrangements, the development of joint research projects and an increase in scope for voluntary sector involvement in interventions with vulnerable populations (WHO 2004: 66). For supporters of the voluntary sector, it is important to find ways to overcome the barriers placed before voluntary groups. This may well mean attempting to give the voluntary sector the kind of stability experienced in state health care. It is increasingly the case, particularly in Britain, that the voluntary sector is seen as a potential partner of the state and private sector in the delivery of health care. The Brown government is willing to strike up a coalition between the state, private and voluntary sectors to tackle public health concerns and to target such problems as obesity (DH 2008d). For some health professionals, however, there are distinct limits to what the voluntary sector can provide (see Box 4.2).

Box 4.2 Health professionals on problems with the voluntary sector

Health professionals are sometimes critical of what the voluntary sector can do to improve health services. Health service managers, for example, have pointed out that voluntary groups often provide low level preventative services rather than more pressured and immediate acute care. It is said also that managers in the voluntary sector often feel unable to evaluate and monitor their services in a thorough manner (Burman et al. 2002: 656). It has been noted also that fundraising often takes place on a local level and is particularly successful in affluent areas. If this method was relied upon too much to raise money for health care initiatives, it could add to the problem of health inequalities (BMA 2002: 29). Kirk (2004) argues that the voluntary sector should be involved in enhancing services rather than undermining what is provided by the state. We should note that health care workers could view the voluntary sector as a form of competition or even as health care by amateurs.

Policy developments

The voluntary sector has something to offer a variety of people through running playgroups, youth clubs and environmental projects or through providing a range of interesting and sometimes offbeat educational courses. In many ways, we look to the voluntary sector to provide those things that the state does not provide or the private sector avoids because they are deemed to be unprofitable. In order to illustrate the developing importance of the voluntary sector in health care, we will look at a few key areas of voluntary sector activity. Voluntary groups have been particularly influential in the development of services for the elderly and for those with mental health problems. Pressures to de-institutionalize geriatric patients and those with mental health problems have created a real need for alternative ways to deliver care. We will touch on these areas when discussing the voluntary sector in Britain, the United States and in other areas of the world.

Britain

The importance of the voluntary sector in Britain, especially in the fields of community care and mental health care, should not be underestimated. Without the voluntary sector, community care initiatives would lack the necessary foundations. Community care has been described as a system of non-state provision aimed particularly at vulnerable or dependant people that takes place in the community in the hope that 'the lives of dependent people are normalized and their contribution to society is valued' (Peckham and Meerabeau 2007: 155). A number of governments in the post-war period argued that community care might provide an answer to the problems of expensive and in many cases dehumanizing care in hospitals. During the mid-1960s, it was argued that community care, consisting mainly of day care services and support in the home of the patient, should be introduced. Although relatively little was done to create the necessary financial and institutional frameworks, governments during the 1970s introduced a series of benefits (most notably Attendance Allowance and Mobility Allowance) in the hope of assisting dependent people who lived in the community. Alongside this, it was argued that dependent people should be encouraged to live normal lives in the community and that this relied upon some provision of informal care. Many of these ideas were formalized in The National Health Service and Community Care Act (NHSCCA 1990) which pushed local authorities away from the direct provision of services towards an 'enabling role' in which they coordinated services provided by the commercial and voluntary sectors. This was viewed by many as an attempt to cut costs and to transfer responsibility for elderly relatives and people with disabilities onto family members (Ackers and Abbott 1996; Perkins 1999; Peckham and Meerabeau 2007). Community care initiatives can create problems for health professionals (see Box 4.3).

Box 4.3   Health professionals on the problems with community care

Community care initiatives were designed to break down at least some of the barriers between patients and the health service. Although this might seem to be a good thing in itself, it has created some issues for health professionals. Nurses have sometimes found that working in the community can lead to a number of problems, especially those of getting too close or too involved with patients. It has been argued that this problem can be minimized by moving nurses around in a team and that this can help nurses to maintain some professional distance (McGarry 2003: 429). It would appear that in devising patient-focussed policies it is important to find a suitable balance between patients and health care professionals. Although patients might prefer to see the same person throughout their treatment, in the case of chronic illness this treatment can extend over a long period however, and unintentionally undermine the position of health care workers.

Party perspectives on community care

The principles of community care have had widespread support from the main political parties in Britain for over forty years. The Labour Party (1964) called for the expansion of domiciliary services (services in the home) to help the elderly and called for increased state regulation of these services. Labour looked for ways to support elderly people who wanted to remain in their homes and favoured supported housing as an alternative to large institutions for those who were unable to live independently (Labour Party 1966). The Labour Party

(1979) claimed that the emphasis should be shifted away from hospital care to care in the community. This move was thought to rely upon strengthening links between social services, health centres and family practitioners. In 1992, the Labour Party promised to appoint a new Minister of State for Community Care with the remit of designing services in line with the demands of the public. This would include increasing the resources available to care for people in their homes and to improving the condition of residential homes (Labour Party 1992).

The Conservative Party has likewise been supportive of care in the community. The Conservative Party (1964) called for an increase in resources to assist the elderly to stay in their own homes rather than be admitted into hospitals. This meant increasing expenditure on home helps, home nurses and health visitors. According to the Conservative Party (1979), people need to be encouraged to look after their own families and greater reliance should be placed on self-help groups and voluntary sector activity. The Conservative Party promoted community care in its general election manifesto of 1983 (Conservative Party 1983) and was responsible for introducing the National Health Service and Community Care Act in 1990. This act did a great deal to establish and formalize community care in Britain. Families had always taken care of elderly members, often without any support. Now this practice became the subject of government policy.

There is a similar commitment to care in the community from the Liberal/SDP Alliance. The Liberal/SDP Alliance saw that involving the voluntary sector in health care provided a way to refocus health care in the community. Voluntary groups were seen as important in supporting people to cope with caring for family members. This applied in particular to helping those who care for elderly relatives (Liberal/SDP Alliance 1983). For the Liberal/SDP Alliance, community care can only become a reality if real support is given to those who care for family members in their own homes and if such support included a package of benefits for carers (Liberal/SDP Alliance 1987). It would seem that the Liberal/SDP Alliance was aware that caring for family members can be expensive and exhausting. Rather than make a virtue out of each family looking after its own members, the Alliance looked for ways to support people in the choices they make.

The value of community care

The value of voluntary sector groups is seen most clearly in helping people to cope and sometimes recover from long-term physical and mental health problems. It is clear that during periods of acute illness, people turn to medical practitioners in the statutory and private sectors but it is in the period after serious illness that the voluntary sector can contribute most. The Department of Health in Britain notes that the voluntary sector is a particularly important provider of intermediate care and that it provides important rehabilitation and preventative services (DH 2000: 97). The voluntary sector is valued greatly in Britain for its role in mental health services. It has been found that voluntary sector involvement in the healing process can enhance recovery from acute illness and that the voluntary sector can help considerably in articulating patient perspectives and assist in the training of health care professionals (DH 2001b: 57). The work of voluntary sector groups in health promotion has also been commended. Voluntary groups have been particularly good at disseminating online information in the field of mental health. Through concerted campaigns, voluntary groups have challenged discrimination and enhanced the opportunities open to those who suffer from poor mental health. This has involved attempts to reduce the stigmas attached to mental health disorders (DH 1999: 37; DH 2001b: 24, 62). In Scotland, voluntary groups have assisted in developing and implementing mental health policies and have been praised for their work in challenging discrimination, promoting recovery and in helping to prevent suicides (Scottish Executive 2003: 6). Voluntary groups often intervene in the hope of stabilizing their users and preventing the onset of further periods of severe illness. This function is particularly important in the context of the financial pressures upon the NHS.

The United States

The voluntary sector is extremely important in the United States. Whereas in Britain the voluntary sector is used to reduce demands upon the resources of the NHS, in the United States it is particularly important as a safety net for those who do not have adequate insurance to access private health care. Self-help groups in particular are recognized by the government of the United States as valuable in assisting patients in recovery from illness (US Department of Health and Human Services 2004: 19). Voluntary groups have been active in setting up drop-in centres and with teaching client groups the skills necessary to manage these centres. The STAR Programme, for example, provides support in setting up and sustaining self-help groups (US Department of Health and Human Services 2004: 20). As we shall see, voluntary activity seems to fit quite well with the individualist political culture of the United States.

The elderly

Self-help groups do some good work with elderly sections of the community. The day care centres run by self-help groups in the United States are thought to reduce the number of elderly people who are admitted to nursing homes. At these centres, elderly people have access to peer counselling and it is recognized that such counselling can help to tackle depression and the problems surrounding bereavement. Attendance at these day care centres can also help to reduce problems stemming from isolation and equip people with numerous coping mechanisms. It is thought that elderly people in particular are uncomfortable with seeking support from the government and that aid provided by their peers is far easier to accept (US Public Health Service 1999: 379; US Department of Health and Human Services 2005b: 24–34). As with many other political cultures, the ethos of self-help is seen as preferable to what could be regarded as accepting handouts from the government.

Mental health

Voluntary groups have also made a major contribution to mental health services in the United States. It has been argued that these services need ethnic minority groups to be involved in recruiting and training people from ethnic minority backgrounds and for developing training on the impact of ethnicity on mental health and accessing services. It is seen as important to develop collaborative relationships with ethnic minority groups to ensure that recovery programmes are developed in a culturally appropriate manner. Indeed, collaborative measures are seen as essential to engage with ethnic minority groups (President's New Freedom Commission on Mental Health 2003: 52–3). In the United States, faith groups work in communities consistently to challenge stigmas associated with poor mental health and to provide support, encourage treatment for depression and identify when a person is at risk. Along with other voluntary sector groups, they work with people in a community setting and require access to suitable training in mental health issues (US Department of Health and Human Services 2001: 54, 80). In the United States, voluntary sector groups were part of a planning team responsible for developing the Surgeon General's Report on Mental Health in 1999. The National Alliance for the Mentally Ill has been particularly influential in its campaigns to expand mental health provision in America (US Public Health Service 1999: 93). Voluntary groups were also involved in the writing and implementation of an important Suicide Prevention Strategy (US Department of Health and Human Services 2001: 21). The American government seems aware of the need to engage constructively with the voluntary sector and to ensure that the services provided take into account the diverse backgrounds, lifestyles and values of those who use the service.

International comparisons

The voluntary sector makes significant contributions to health care, especially in those countries with limited welfare states. As we have seen when discussing voluntary activity in the United States, the voluntary sector can be viewed as a preferred alternative to state intervention. Many countries rely upon informal care. This applies in particular to caring for elderly relatives where the obligation or burden of care often falls upon women. It has been noted that the responsibility of families for care is emphasized heavily in Germany, Japan and Singapore. In Germany, for example, the state is only meant to intervene in the last resort if families or the voluntary sector have failed to provide adequate care (Blank and Bureau 2004). Although voluntary sector intervention in social care is regarded with less disdain than state intervention, it is still seen as inferior to the obligations we have to our own families.

Supplementing services

The voluntary sector is also important to the welfare regimes of countries with well-developed welfare states. We have seen that Britain has turned increasingly towards using the voluntary sector as the state has attempted to relinquish some of its social responsibilities. The same process seems to have taken place in Canada and in Sweden. In Canada, self-help groups provide important emotional support and mutual aid especially in the field of mental health (Tramior et al. 2004: 8). In Sweden, the traditional reliance upon the state was undermined during the 1990s and replaced with an increase in service delivery by voluntary groups (Blank and Bureau 2004). It would appear that many of these state-centred welfare regimes have recognized that using the voluntary sector for some service delivery, especially in preventative and rehabilitation work, might help to protect state health care from the pressures of excessive demand.

The only alternative

We should not forget, moreover, that the voluntary sector is sometimes all that is available. This applies in particular to mental health provision. In many parts of central and eastern Europe, the state has been unwilling to provide adequate mental health services. This has created a vacuum, which has been filled to some extent by voluntary groups particularly in Hungary, Lithuania, Romania and Slovakia (European Commission 2006: 86, 106, 137 and 143). In the developing world, the voluntary sector has been left to deliver essential mental health services. In India, for example, the Schizophrenia Research Foundation is one of the most important providers of mental health services (WHO 2003: 6, 41). In these countries, where economic pressures would appear to be acute, the voluntary sector helps to make up for the lack of affordable health care and for the apparent disengagement of the state from certain areas of health care.

Conclusion

The voluntary sector does tremendous work in helping communities to help themselves. It is recognized that the voluntary sector is well placed to intervene in the community and to be sensitive in its dealings with marginalized groups. The voluntary sector often works far better than the state with these groups. This could be because the state is limited in scope when it attempts to provide a standardized service regardless of the particular needs of different parts of the community. The voluntary sector is praised for its innovative and committed workforce, but often faces instability in funding and in the career paths offered to its workers. Governments can help by providing sustainable core funding, but it is quite evident that voluntary groups have to think freshly about their aims to match the changing priorities advanced by funding bodies. Supporters of state health care recognize that the voluntary sector can help to relieve pressure on the statutory sector, while supporters of the private sector consider these community groups preferable to dependence upon the state. There is, of course, a limit to what the voluntary sector can provide. Voluntary groups are often staffed by community workers and by volunteers who often have limited opportunities for training rather than by trained health care professionals. This can create some tensions between the sectors and some obstacles to effective collaboration between the voluntary sector, the state and the private sector. It should be recognized, however, that the voluntary sector offers a useful supplement to state and private sector health care and is particularly important in intermediate and community care. Taken together, the state, the private sector and the voluntary sector represent the main participants in a mixed economy of care and a range of alternatives available to those engaged in the development of health policy.

PART 2
SETTING PRIORITIES

5   Health inequalities

Chapter Contents

We live in an unequal society. If you turn on a television set and flick randomly through the channels you will be subjected to a dramatic array of lifestyles. Walk through any city in the West and you will move through areas of relative prosperity and those of relative deprivation. Many people who study for a degree do so in the hope that it will help them secure a place in society of reasonable security and comfort. It is unusual to encounter a student studying for a degree who aspires to live in poverty and who accepts that they will be unable to access the health care they need when they need it. Yet we are surrounded by inequalities in health care. Just as individuals have health care needs, so too do social groups. People from different classes, genders and ethnic groups will tend to have different health care needs.

This chapter considers and discusses the ways to help answer the following questions:

- To what extent should the state attempt to alleviate inequalities in health?
- Does it matter that some groups have better health than others?
- Should there be a system of positive discrimination in health care in which the health care needs of deprived groups are given greater priority than the health care needs of the prosperous?

- Do health care professionals need to concern themselves with such things?
- If the answer to this final question is yes, then what can be done?

Health care professionals within many Western societies will work within diverse and unequal communities. It would be unrealistic for somebody training to be a health professional to assume that they will only ever treat people from their own class, gender, age and ethnic background. People will have different needs and perhaps part of being a health care professional involves being able to identify and respond to these differences. According to Hausman et al. (2002) it is important for health professionals to understand health inequalities because it can add to their understanding of the causes of good and bad health. It is also important to understand health inequalities because such inequalities might stem from and lead to other injustices. They claim that if health is indeed influenced by social factors, then it is possible to challenge health inequalities through a series of social policy initiatives. As we shall see, there are many ways in which governments can respond to health inequalities. This chapter is concerned in part with outlining some of the innovative ways in which health policies have attempted to tackle health inequalities. But first we take a look at some of the arguments for and against the state intervening to reduce these inequalities.

Theoretical perspectives

What does it matter if one group of people has better health than another? We should be aware that inequality in itself is not always seen as a social ill. We are surrounded by inequalities. There are physical inequalities in terms of the strength that we have at our disposal. The capitalist economy positively encourages economic inequalities. They are seen as being good to spur people on to succeed, accumulate material wealth and to elevate their social standing. There are cultural inequalities, stemming perhaps from our educational background and achievements, the books we read, the music we listen to and the television we watch. Although many of these inequalities are the result of the decisions we have made, they also have a lot to do with our class background, the dominant sub-cultures in our communities and the opinions and aspirations of family and friends. The arguments made for and against tackling health inequalities have to take into account these broader social factors. We should appreciate that the health we have and the ways in which we choose to manage our own health will be influenced by the income at our disposal, the quality of our homes and neighbourhoods, our educational background and social circumstances. Few would argue that our social surroundings have no impact upon our health. The question is not whether social factors have an influence upon health but whether the state has an obligation to tackle inequalities in general and health inequalities in particular.

Arguments in support of tackling health inequalities

Arguments in favour of the state intervening to tackle health inequalities could be developed from social democratic foundations. Social democrats tend to favour the building of a more equal society. Because of this, they support the redistribution of both wealth and of opportunities. This could include investing in state schools, programmes of social housing or tending to the health needs of vulnerable or at risk groups in society. If we were to follow the logic of social democratic arguments, the state should invest more resources in health care in poorer areas. For some commentators, this makes perfect sense. Boseley (2002) believes that tackling health inequalities can help the NHS to save money in the long run and that, if the health status of the poorest sections of the community could be raised to the same level as the affluent sections, hospital admissions could be cut by about 6 per cent per year and thus secure a saving of about $850 million per year (Boseley 2002: 5). Rob Baggott (2000) likewise argues that health policy should look into improving living and working conditions to help prevent inequalities developing and to create a level playing field for all. Some groups will almost inevitably fall through the net and not take advantage of opportunities presented to them, but this should not stand in the way of people being consulted on their health needs and participating in decision making on health. According to this line of thought, we need to devise holistic strategies to tackle inequalities in health. Those who believe that the state should intervene to tackle health inequalities are well aware that this relies not only upon the actions of good intentioned medics but also upon a broader social programme in which in which all forms of inequality are addressed.

The importance of social policies

So what kind of policies should be pursued? Drawing upon research conducted by the Kings Fund, Benzaval and Judge (1995) pointed out that health inequalities should be attacked using a broad range of social policies. In particular, they supported state intervention in housing, employment and in health promotion. They argued that the state should invest more in social housing and that it was possible to use community regeneration schemes to make significant improvements to the environment and to the local economic and social systems. State intervention in creating sustainable employment opportunities could be focussed on education and training, expanding childcare facilities and upon reforming the benefits system to help low paid workers. In their view, it was also necessary for the state to move away from blaming the victims of poor health and to recognize that health damaging behaviour often stems from people having to cope with poor living conditions. In their view, the state should be more involved in promoting good health (Benzaval and Judge 1995). The policy recommendations outlined above show how tackling health inequalities should be seen in the context of a comprehensive programme of social policies. If governments intervene to improve levels of health, this should help to reduce costs of acute care and perhaps reduce levels of dependence upon welfare benefits. Although extensive social programmes might appear to be quite expensive, there are certainly long-term gains to be had.

A question of priorities

A comprehensive programme of social policies, however, might be too expensive to implement. If health inequalities are to be tackled, especially in the context of limited resources, it might be necessary to prioritize some things over others. But how could these priorities be set? According to Black and Mooney (2002), it is unrealistic to expect the health system to achieve full equality of health care, given the vast range of personal factors that influence our health. What is important, however, is that there is at least equal funding per capita and that due attention is given to the problems faced by disadvantaged communities (Black and Mooney 2002: 194). Graham and Kelly (2004) believe that attention should be paid to relative disadvantage and that attempts must be made to narrow the gap between classes and groups in society. Concentrating upon differentials in health status is deemed more important because it can help to widen the scope of policy interventions. Such intervention would be more inclusive and it would deal with the majority of the population rather than concentrate solely upon the welfare of the bottom layer (Graham and Kelly 2004: 2–10). According to this line of thought, tackling health inequalities does not necessarily mean improving the health of the poor especially when this is at the expense of other classes in society. Instead, health inequalities between all social classes need to be addressed. If it is indeed possible to develop a more inclusive approach, this could increase levels of public support for such measures and thereby reduce possible resistance from less disadvantaged sections of society.

Scenario 10 Tackling health inequalities

Sarah is a young single mother who lives on a council estate with her newborn baby. She is suffering from post-natal depression and has poor social networks. Her health visitor has tried to encourage her to attend a group for mothers and babies and to seek advice from her GP. Sarah, however, has no means of transport and little spare money for bus fares. She lives in an area with a high crime rate and is afraid to walk very far. From part of the funding for the mother and baby group, a taxi is arranged to take Sarah to group meetings.

Questions

You are a health care worker working in Sarah's community:

1 To what extent and in what ways is Sarah's health being adversely affected by her socio-economic circumstances?
2 What else, if anything, could be done to help Sarah?

Arguments against tackling health inequalities

The case against tackling health inequalities rests upon the belief that each of us is responsible for our own level of health and that the state has no real responsibility to remedy such inequalities. This is consistent with a neo-liberal world view in which individuals are urged to pursue their own interests without being shackled by the high levels of taxation needed to implement egalitarian policies. The Conservative governments of 1979–1997, under the leadership of Margaret Thatcher (1979–1990) and John Major (1990–1997), saw very little need to assume responsibility for challenging inequalities in health. Although these governments were provided with evidence (most notably from the Black Report of 1980) that there were definite links between class and health and there had been an increase in the difference in mortality rates between the classes, the Conservative governments chose to ignore these findings in favour of blaming the victims of poor health for living unhealthy lifestyles (see Webster 1998: 137). From a neo-liberal point of view, individuals need to dedicate themselves to improving their own health rather than rely upon the government providing extra resources to ease the way.

The third way

Existing somewhere between the views that the responsibility for tackling health inequalities rest with the state (a social democratic view) or the individual (a neo-liberal view) is the so-called 'third way' approach that promises resources to help individuals improve their own health. This approach to health inequalities is enshrined within the theoretical perspectives and policy developments inaugurated by the British Labour Party since 1997. The Labour government (DH 2004a) claimed that people, especially those in disadvantaged areas, should be encouraged to make healthy choices and that it was important to target 'communities and groups where opportunities to choose health are less developed and most progress is needed' (DH 2004a: 14). The Labour government, however, rejected the view that this is a one-way process in which the government assumes ultimate responsibility and provides all of the necessary resources. John Reid, the former Health Secretary, was adamant that the government can do very little to reduce health inequalities unless disadvantaged people also work towards overcoming the conditions that make them disadvantaged (Reid 2004). Within this approach, there are clear signs that individuals are to be made accountable for their own health but that help is available to those who seek to improve their own health.

Scenario 11 Tackling health inequalities

Let us return to Sarah, a single mother with post-natal depression, poor social networks, limited financial resources and living in an area with a high crime rate. Here are two other ways to view partial solutions to her circumstances.

a   The health visitor suggests that she asks her family for help and talks to her about some self-help techniques to combat her depression.
b   The health visitor encourages Sarah to get involved in a new community project to tackle the problems of local crime.

Questions

Take a look at the advice given by the health visitor:

1   To what extent do you feel that these pieces of advice are useful?
2   How does the advice given correspond to the theoretical perspectives outlined in this chapter?

Policy developments

Policies that aim to address health inequalities have had to deal with a range of problems facing different sections of the community. It must surely be the case that policies focussing upon reducing inequalities between classes will not necessarily do anything in themselves to close the gap between different genders or ethnic groups. As we will see, each particular section of the community has its own needs which give rise to different policy responses.

Britain

The attempt to tackle and reduce health inequalities is associated in particular with the ideas and policies of the Labour Party. As we saw in the section on theoretical perspectives, social democrats are committed to reducing all types of inequality whereas neo-liberals tend to believe that this would be messing with the natural order of things. The Labour Party, which has been heavily influenced by social democratic ideas for much of its history, has targeted health inequalities in its policy proposals. In 1983, the Labour Party pledged to reduce inequalities in access to health care and to ensure that resources were placed into primary health care facilities in inner city areas (see Labour Party 1983). In 1992 the Labour Party promised to set up a new National Health Initiative to promote physical and mental health and to reduce health inequalities between classes and ethnic groups (Labour Party 1992). Although the ideological complexion of the Labour Party changed with the development of New Labour and the third way, the Labour Party has remained convinced that health policies should be formulated to reduce health inequalities.

Facing the problem of health inequalities

When the Labour Party returned to power in 1997 it pledged immediate support to tackling the problem of health inequalities. It was acknowledged that this task required the active cooperation of different government departments and entailed dealing with problems in education, employment, housing and social care (DH 1997). The Labour government set up an enquiry under Donald Acheson to investigate the problem of health inequalities. The aim of the Acheson enquiry was not merely to identify the extent of health inequalities but also to suggest some solutions. Acheson (1998) noted that although there had been improvements in general levels of health in Britain since the formation of the NHS, inequalities in health had increased; so much so that it made sense for any government committed to undermining health inequalities to identify key priorities and divert resources to where they were needed (Acheson 1998). For those who believe that the government should intervene in this way, it is not a matter of attempting to throw more money at all health problems but of targeting particular groups of people and attempting to improve their level of health. Acheson (1998) suggested that the NHS should work with a variety of agencies in tackling health inequalities. These agencies included:

- local authorities;
- groups involved in community regeneration projects;
- voluntary sector groups;
- the business community.

These groups could help in financing and running a variety of projects. It was felt, for example, they might have a role in the building of healthy living centres in poorer areas and that these centres could help to improve the health of some disadvantaged groups (Acheson 1998). This enquiry helped to set the tone for Labour policy on health inequalities since 1997.

Labour policy on health inequalities

The Labour government was convinced that people suffered from poor health because of a range of social problems relating to standard of living, quality of life, housing, education, employment and so on. If health inequalities were to be dealt with, then the solution required some 'joined up' thinking. Resources were increased for primary care and health visitors went out into the community to assess the extent of health problems and to work with families to improve levels of health (see Appleby 1997; Graham 1997; Webster 1998; Abercrombie and Warde 2000). The health secretary John Reid pointed out that the Labour government believes that inequalities in health can only be tackled through multi-agency work and that it is important to involve different government departments, the NHS, voluntary and community groups and local government (Reid 2004: 3). This emphasis upon working in the communities became an important feature of Labour policy and has had a dramatic impact upon the work undertaken by health professionals (see Box 5.1).

Box 5.1   Nurses, health inequalities and the community

Nurses have an increasingly important role in the fight against health inequalities. By working in the community, district nurses in Britain have become important agents of change and key participants in the development of local health initiatives (Nursing in Practice 2006). Through their work with children and parents, school nurses have also been able to exert an influence upon lifestyle choices and thus help to reduce health-damaging behaviour. Nurses have been urged to increase their role in community development work in the belief that this will allow them to reach a broader group of people (Winters et al. 2007). It is clear that nurses can have a dramatic impact upon the lives and health of members of the community, though this influence requires nurses to be socially engaged. Rather than see their role as being to assist other health care professionals (doctors in particular), nurses can enhance their position and influence by taking on work in the community and by expanding their work to include communicating with different groups of people about their health.

The Labour government in Britain has been particularly active in its campaign to lessen health inequalities. It has stated that the existence of wide inequalities in health is unacceptable and that governments should be willing to put resources into narrowing the disparity and inequality in the health status of different groups. The Health Inequalities Unit in the Department of Health aims to reduce health inequalities by 10 per cent by 2010. These inequalities are measured according to infant mortality and life expectancy (DH 2008a). In Scotland, a system of positive discrimination has been introduced to reduce the incidence of poor health among deprived sections of the community. It is recognized, however, that there are significant barriers to reaching deprived groups and widespread reluctance to change behaviour among some groups. Because of this, health promotion campaigns are often less effective in Scotland (Medical Research Council 2007). A multi-agency approach is used to address the problems of social exclusion. Special emphasis is placed upon developing early intervention strategies and making primary care more proactive (Scottish Executive 2006b). We should be aware, however, that different groups in society suffer from poor health and that strategies designed for one group will not necessarily be successful in dealing with the problems faced by another group. Let us take a closer look at these groups.

Class

Social exclusion of all sorts can have a negative impact upon health. The collapse of traditional industries, for example, has left some communities with few options and little hope. The experience of unemployment can be particularly dramatic and have devastating effects on health. It has been found that middle-aged men who are made unemployed are at greater risk of premature death than those who remain in work. Unemployed people are also more likely to experience neurotic symptoms than those in work (Baggott 2000: 229). Social exclusion disempowers people and can make them prone to higher levels of stress and to lower levels of self esteem (Davis 1999: 137). When we talk about the impact of social exclusion on health, we are not simply referring to a few isolated individuals who have hit upon hard times. Social exclusion often affects entire communities, especially those facing economic decline because of the closure of local businesses. People with poor health often find it difficult to find and hold onto well paid jobs. Those from poorer sections of the community are also more likely to smoke and to place less emphasis upon regular exercise. Poor nutrition, poor living conditions and environmental pollution can also exacerbate these problems (Davis 1999; Alcock et al. 2000: 207–8; Baggott 2000: 226–7). Economic problems can thus set off a chain reaction and drag down both individuals and communities.

It is important to realize that poverty is *relative*. Although the majority of the poorer sections of Britain experience better health now than the poor before the Second World War, the gap is still considerable between the classes. The poor suffer from *relative material deprivation*. Their health has improved, but so has the health of higher socio-economic classes. Because of this, health inequalities remain (Gillespie and Prior 1995: 204). Poverty can have a devastating effect because it touches all parts of the lives of its victims. It impacts upon levels of income, housing and nutrition as well as upon general levels of mental health (Shaw et al. 1999: 216). The environment in which we live often influences the health we experience. This applies in particular, though not exclusively, to the housing we occupy. Poor housing can have an extremely detrimental effect upon health. Respiratory problems can arise from damp living conditions and overcrowding can increase levels of stress and accidents in the home (Baggott 2000: 229). These economic and social factors need to be taken into account when attempting to deal with class inequalities in health.

The existence of class inequalities in health has been recognized for some time. Titmus (1968) noted that inequalities in health continued and he believed that this was partly because people from higher income groups tend to be more adept at accessing resources and obtaining specialist treatment. More recent government reports have acknowledged that class inequalities in health are particularly difficult to reduce or remove. The Department of Health (DH 2005c) claims that people from poor backgrounds tend to feel less in control of their circumstances and might thus have more difficulty in making healthy choices. If class inequalities in health are to be tackled, then something must surely be done to address the problems of class inequality as a whole. Acheson (1998) was adamant that solutions needed to include a commitment to improve the health of young mothers and women of child-bearing age. The benefits system, pensions and employment policies also required a general overhaul so as to improve the economic and social prospects of poorer sections of the community. The Brown government continued to support active intervention in primary health care to tackle the problems of health inequalities and to deal with at least some of the disadvantages experienced by those who live in relatively poor conditions (DH 2008d). In Scotland, attempts have been made to close the 'opportunity gap' through tackling low income, lack of opportunities and aspirations and through attempting to undermine factors that prevented people from participating fully in society (Scottish Executive 2006a). Tackling class inequalities in health has relied upon targeting the problems stemming from social exclusion and raising awareness among health professionals (see Box 5.2).

Box 5.2 Health professionals on class inequalities

When dealing with patients, it is important to take into consideration their social circumstances and their cultural values. The social circumstances of patients can make them more prone to certain types of illness and their cultural values can influence the degree to which they are successful in gaining access to appropriate services. Being sensitive towards the impact of class upon health can help health care workers in their relationships with patients. The Royal College of Radiologists (2005) calls upon its members to recognize the impact of social class upon health and upon accessing services. While recognizing that some of these inequalities are systemic and related to other types of inequality, radiologists are urged to search for ways to minimize their impact upon the care they provide. The Royal College of Radiologists claims, moreover, that understanding health inequalities should be included within the training that radiologists receive.

Gender

Although women on average have longer lives than men, women tend to suffer from poorer health than men. When we think about health inequalities, therefore, we should take into account differences between genders. Acheson (1998) identified a number of ways that gender inequalities in health could be reduced. The problem of death from traffic accidents, especially involving young men, could be alleviated through further interventions to prevent and penalize speeding. Suicide rates among men could also be tackled through improving opportunities for work. Psycho-social illnesses experienced by young women, especially those caring for young children, could be approached by providing good quality social housing and by investing in health visitors to work with young mothers. The poor health experienced by many older women could be improved through increased investment in housing, measures to reduce the fear of crime and through concessions on public transport (see Acheson 1998). Policy makers in Britain have become increasingly aware of the different ways in which men and women view their own health and treat themselves. Recent priorities in health promotion work have included tackling obesity, mental health problems, Coronary Heart Disease, sexual health, cancer and alcohol abuse. In each case, perceived differences between the genders have been used in the development of suitable interventions (DH 2008c). The Brown government was particularly keen on targeting middle-aged men and helping to keep them in work. Health 'MOTs' have been designed to detect health problems stemming from health damaging behaviour in the hope of reducing the number of heart attacks, strokes and incidence of diabetes (DH 2008d). Solutions to health inequalities are often couched within a broader framework of interventions in the economy and society. For health professionals this often means working closely with patients in the community (see Box 5.3).

Box 5.3   Health professionals on health inequalities and women

In addressing health inequalities, it is important that health care workers are aware of the need for long-term developmental work with their patients. Health inequalities can not usually be eradicated through a single intervention but will often require a series of measures, delivered over time. Midwives have been urged to work closely with women in the community in an attempt to reduce health inequalities. Midwives have become far more involved with smoking cessation and with attempting to reduce levels of teenage pregnancy (Smith 2005b). This shows that the role of a midwife goes far beyond supporting women in childbirth and includes a much broader community remit. This will also apply to other health care professionals. The task of combating gender inequalities in health should not fall solely to those who deal primarily with women. It is surely something that all health care workers can embrace.

Ethnic minorities

Ethnic minority groups can also face a series of problems that damage their health. Reid and Phillips (2004) argue that the approach traditionally taken by the Labour Party to address health inequalities has been to emphasize the importance of uniformity of provision and that this has failed to give sufficient weight to diversity in society. Patients from ethnic minority backgrounds often encounter difficulties when they access primary health care facilities. Acheson (1998) states that problems can arise because there might be:

- communication difficulties if the patient's first language is not English. Chinese people, for example, have had particular problems understanding their GPs;
- cultural differences in the way that symptoms are described;
- cultural differences with regard to gender issues. Pakistani women, for example, often prefer to be treated by women from the same background.

Cultural differences can account for at least some of the inequalities in health. There tend to be higher rates of smoking found among African Caribbean and Bangladeshi men and lower rates of physical exercise among Indian, Bangladeshi and Pakistani men (Baggott 2000: 233). Research has revealed the existence of high levels of poverty among ethnic minorities. This applies in particular to Caribbean, Pakistani and Bangladeshi families (see Abercrombie and Warde 2000). We should remember that these social factors do not operate in isolation. A person might be poor and from an ethnic minority background.

According to Acheson (1998), solutions to these problems might involve training health care workers to be sensitive to cultural differences and to understand that people from different cultures will often use different terms to describe an illness. The profile and status of ethnic minority patients can also be enhanced through making translators available and by recruiting health care workers from diverse backgrounds. Involving ethnic minority groups in decision-making bodies can help to educate health care practitioners in cultural diversity and serve to reduce feelings of isolation and powerlessness. The health inequalities suffered by ethnic minority groups therefore can only be addressed to the extent that health care professionals and facilities are willing to take into account the needs of diverse communities and recognize that one size does not fit all.

The United States

Despite differences in political culture and the role of the state in health care, approaches to reducing health inequalities in the United States are remarkably similar to the approaches taken in Britain. The New York City Department of Health and Mental Hygiene (2004), for example, recognizes the impact of economic and social factors on health. It has proposed that health inequalities should be tackled through:

- the development of preventative health care;
- the promotion of healthy lifestyles;
- the creation of better environmental conditions;
- concerted attacks against poverty.

It has argued that addressing health inequalities requires substantial investment in housing, education, the leisure industry and the economy and it has been involved in promoting regular health checks and in a variety of strategies to reduce dependence upon alcohol, tobacco and drugs. The logic is clear. If the state of our health is influenced by economic and social factors then the solutions to poor health need to include a selection of economic and social policies.

Class

Health authorities in the United States have identified some of the ways that economic and cultural status can impact upon health. It is claimed that people from disadvantaged backgrounds are more likely to suffer from obesity, diabetes and heart disease. Those from privileged backgrounds, on the other hand, often experience better health as a result of living in safer areas, in better housing and through accessing superior health care (US Department of Health and Human Services 2000b). The extent of the problem varies considerably across the United States. It is estimated that 21 per cent of people in New York live below the poverty line compared with a national average of 12 per cent. Poor housing, low levels of community cohesion and high levels of crime are all thought to increase stress and anxiety and have a negative impact upon health in New York (New York City Department of Health and Mental Hygiene 2004). The solution to class inequalities in health is thought to lie in a series of economic and social interventions. According to the US Department of Health and Human Services (2000b), interventions should take place in education, housing, transport and community safety.

Gender

Gender inequalities in health are not high on the political agenda in the United States. More often than not, greater attention is paid to the problems affecting those who are either economically disadvantaged or an ethnic minority. Some states have their own departments for women's health. In New York, for example, there are some women's health programmes that deal in particular with family planning and sexual health (see New York State Department of Health 2004) but these measures tend to be quite localized and do not appear to be part of a national or federal strategy.

Ethnic minorities

There are a number of factors that contribute towards poor levels of health among ethnic minority groups in the United States. It has been noted (see Institute of Medicine 2002) that ethnic minority patients sometimes encounter prejudice and bias in their dealings with health care providers and that ethnic minorities receive less care, delay seeking care, are believed to comply poorly with treatment and mistrust health care professionals. According to the Institute of Medicine (2002), solutions to ethnic inequalities in health in the United States should include cross-cultural education in which health care workers are encouraged to develop sensitivity towards other cultures, skills in dealing with diverse groups and effective ways to communicate with different groups. These solutions to health inequalities focus primarily upon what health care professionals can do to adapt their services to the needs of ethnic minority groups and to address the bad reputation that health care providers have among these sections of the community.

International comparisons

The need to deal with health inequalities is recognized in many parts of the world. Throughout the European Union, attempts are being made to reduce inequalities in health. In France, health promotion strategies focus upon early childhood in particular in an attempt to reduce long-term inequalities in health. Regional networks have been established in Germany to tackle disparities in health, while in Belgium a national body has been established to coordinate local initiatives aimed particularly at improving the health of vulnerable groups (European Commission 2007). Countries with well-developed systems of state health care have been at the forefront of attempts to undermine health inequalities. This has applied to inequalities based upon class, ethnicity and gender.

Class

Attempts to tackle class inequalities in health have attained increasing importance in Canada. The Canadian government has been committed to tackling health inequalities since 2002 when a series of initiatives were launched to improve the health of vulnerable sections of the community and to bridge the gap between the community and providers of primary health care (Health

Disparities Task Group of the Federal/Provincial/Territorial Advisory Committee on Population Health and Health Security 2004). Recommendations for redressing inequalities in health include making improvements to levels of literacy, education, income and benefits for low income families (Canadian Population Health Initiative 2004). Economic tools have been used to address disparities in health. By attempting to increase employment opportunities, enhancing the benefits available for the elderly and for families raising children and through increasing investment in education, the Canadian government has signalled its commitment to a fairer and less divided society and to improving the health of all citizens (Canadian Population Health Initiative 2004). It is important to note that tackling health inequalities does not necessarily mean that resources are shifted from the affluent to the poor. Health interventions in poor communities could indeed reduce pressures upon state health care and thereby benefit all sections of the community. It is sometimes more a case of changing the focus of intervention rather than increasing the total amount. Shifting some resources into health promotion, for example, can lead to savings in other parts of a state funded health service.

Gender
Approaches to gender inequalities in health vary considerably across the world. In Sweden, there is no attempt to divide the genders and develop separate policies. Health policy is developed as an integrated package to apply to all citizens equally (see Swedish National Institute of Public Health 2008). This approach, which relies upon developing inclusive services, is not favoured by all countries.

If health systems are to address inequalities, then another approach can be used in which the different genders are targeted. Acknowledging that men and women approach health in different ways, the Canadian government recognizes that there will be differences in how men and women respond to health promotion campaigns. Considerable resources have been dedicated to promoting women's health and to advancing awareness of women's health needs. The development of health policy in Canada has made extensive use of gender based analysis as a research tool to investigate the impact of policy initiatives on men and women and to further understanding of the impact of gender upon health (see Status of Women in Canada 1995; Health Canada 1999; Health Canada 2003). In Australia, attempts to improve the health of women have tended to focus upon women who are marginalized or isolated because of their geographical location, ethnic background or because of economic deprivation. This work has included addressing some of the main barriers to these women in accessing appropriate health care. Sometimes the barriers are cultural, other times they are economic. The Australian government does recognize, however, that the health services available need to be made more flexible and sensitive to the needs of marginalized groups of women (Department of Health and Ageing 2008b).

Governments have also recognized that the health needs of men require attention. In Australia and New Zealand, policy makers have concentrated upon improving the health of men. In Australia, there has been some concern over the number of industrial accidents involving men and attempts have been made to improve levels of health care and other support packages for men from indigenous communities (Human Rights and Equal Opportunities Commission 2008). In New Zealand, campaigns have been developed to increase the awareness of men of their own health and health needs and to encourage men to take advantage of health checks (Ministry of Health 2008). Anecdotal evidence suggests that men are notoriously bad at monitoring their own health and in accessing suitable support. This is something that the architects of health policy and health promotion campaigns need to be aware of.

Ethnic minorities

The health inequalities affecting different ethnic minority groups are of international concern. The Dutch government, for example, has become acutely aware of the need to curb inequalities in health care in general and to improve the health levels of the ethnic minority population in particular. Ten per cent of the Dutch population are from an ethnic minority background so interventions have to be developed to cater for a large number of people. The Dutch government has called for funded initiatives to increase awareness of cultural diversity, more reliable information for ethnic minorities on the workings of the Dutch health care system and an expansion in the training given to health care professionals on ethnicity and its impact upon health (see Olthuis and Van Heteren 2003). This approach bears some resemblance to that used in Britain and the United States. In each case, the solutions to ethnic inequalities in health are seen in the context of the standard state health care system. It relies upon making health care workers more aware of different needs and informing ethnic minority groups of their rights to, and the benefits of, health care.

The problems facing ethnic minority groups and health care providers are sometimes not easily accommodated within standard provision. It is sometimes necessary to provide an alternative service. This would seem to apply in both Canada and Australia. According to the Canadian Population Health Initiative (2004), aboriginal health problems in Canada include:

- high levels of injuries (approximately four times greater than the rest of the population);
- high levels of respiratory diseases, attributed to poor housing conditions;

- mental health problems stemming from the erosion of their own language and culture;
- obesity resulting from the decline of their traditional diet.

The Canadian Population Health Initiative (2004) recognizes the need to take a holistic approach when dealing with the health needs of aboriginal people and argues that the aim should be to create a culturally sensitive service based upon the active involvement of aboriginal people.

A similar approach can be seen in Australia. The Australian Institute of Health and Welfare (2006) has noted that over 70 per cent of indigenous Australians die before they are 65 years old compared with a figure of 20 per cent for the rest of the population. Indigenous Australians are disadvantaged in many ways. They tend to have lower incomes, poorer levels of education and lower rates of employment. There are also high levels of dependence on alcohol and drugs. Black and Mooney (2002) believe that it is important for health care professionals to make decisions about treatment based upon the values of the community with which they are dealing rather than in accordance with their own personal (and quite possibly elitist) values. For example, when doctors in Australia treat aboriginal people it is important that they take into account the way that aboriginal people regard themselves in relation to their community. When doctors fail to take this into account, they often find that their interventions are unsuccessful. For this reason, doctors have been urged to be aware of the cultural baggage that people carry and to involve the community in identifying its health care needs (Black and Mooney 2002: 200–5; see also Box 5.4). We should avoid constructing a single template for good and bad health and recognize that it makes far more sense to get an idea of what kind of health people want to achieve for themselves.

Box 5.4   Health inequalities and health training in Australia

Finding ways to increase awareness of health inequalities will always be a problem, especially where formal training is carried out using a bio-medical approach to health. A broader social approach is needed to highlight and to recognize the importance of health inequalities and to point to the relevance of this understanding for professional practice. There are, however, some good examples of training in which social factors are given due weight. GPs in Australia, for example, are expected as part of their training to study and deal with the impact of economic and social deprivation upon health. The academic curricula for GPs include modules on the social context of health and they are also subjected to diverse health care needs in their placements (Furler et al. 2007).

Conclusion

If we are to determine the extent to which the state should be involved in reducing health inequalities, we need to take into account a range of economic and social issues. It makes little sense to argue that health inequalities should be removed if we are not also willing to invest in other areas of the economy and society. As we have seen, health inequalities stem not only from lifestyle choices but also from one's class, gender and ethnicity. This list is by no means complete. Age could certainly be added, as could the type of work we do and a multitude of other factors. By looking at class, gender and ethnicity, we have been able to identify some of the ways our social identities impact upon our health and some of the solutions to health inequalities offered by a variety of health services. Common to many of these policy agendas is the belief that the services available have to take into account the needs of different groups and that health care professionals require a broad social awareness so that they are equipped to deal with the diverse needs and demands of their patients. Tackling health inequalities requires health care professionals to be proactive and work with communities of people suffering from poor health. This work will often involve liaising with other agencies and requires health care professionals to look beyond the surface. Patients are influenced (or even trapped) by their social circumstances. If health inequalities are to be lessened, then these circumstances have to be considered. It is unlikely that private health care providers will have any sustained interest in tackling health inequalities. Campaigns to reduce health inequalities therefore rely to a large extent upon state intervention in the direction and provision of health care and in finding solutions to broader economic and social inequalities. Anything less is merely tinkering with the symptoms and ignoring the problem.

6 Health promotion

Chapter Contents

In discussing modern health systems, it might be tempting to think about those services designed to respond to acute medical needs. We might, for example, have a mental image of a busy hospital ward or a packed waiting room. If we do indeed hold onto these images, any talk about cutting costs and reducing services will undoubtedly be more difficult as we face the realities of these wards or waiting rooms being even busier. But let us not despair. Health promotion provides us with another way to look at health care. Instead of thinking only about responding to illness and acute need, health promotion diverts our attention towards intervening to improve levels of health and possibly reduce demands for acute care. We should be aware, however, that these interventions could be seen as being too intrusive, as a threat to the freedom of the individual and no doubt raise a number of important questions about the freedom to choose one's own lifestyle. This chapter discusses and helps answer questions, such as:

- Should we be free to consume as much alcohol as we like for as long as we like, or does our freedom rely upon us placing limits upon what we drink so that we can develop other interests and skills?
- Are people who smoke thirty or forty cigarettes a day free or are they slaves to their habits?

To those who want the freedom to indulge their habits, health promotion can be seen as a potential threat to the lifestyle decisions they have made for themselves. Knowing this, it would seem important for governments to find ways to communicate and promote their public health messages without alienating those deemed to be most at risk.

Health promotion is generally concerned with finding ways to improve the health of the individual and the community. It goes beyond traditional methods of curing illness and seeks to improve well-being by helping people to live more productive and fulfilling lives (Wall and Owen 1999: 133–4). Although it could be argued that people should be sufficiently mindful of their own well-being to make healthy choices without having to be prompted, this fails to take into account many of the economic, social and environmental factors that shape our health. Simply leaving people to endure poor health would be heartless at best and would neglect to give due weight to the importance of individual health for the general health and well-being of society. It is argued that our levels of health will often be influenced by the choices we make and by the ways in which we take advantage of opportunities for improving our health (see DH 2004). According to this line of thought, the individual is an active agent in the process rather than a passive recipient or beneficiary of a state of health.

There are many strategies used in health promotion. Lifestyle campaigns warn people about such things as the dangers of smoking. The government might also intervene directly to improve the health of the population by regulating levels of pollution or by increasing taxation on harmful substances. There is also a range of preventative measures that can be put in place to improve general levels of health. Primary prevention might include introducing laws to prevent dangerous behaviour. Secondary prevention includes such things as screening services. Tertiary prevention could involve measures to minimize the effects of a disability or to provide extra care for vulnerable sections of the community (Wall and Owen 1999: 134–6). Although health professionals have an important role in health promotion (see Box 6.1), it is unlikely that they can do everything themselves without the cooperation and support of the state. Nordenfelt (2001) argues that the responsibility for health promotion lies outside of the medical professions and that the government must have some involvement in the provision of health-enhancing facilities (like gyms) and in restricting health-damaging activities (like smoking) (Nordenfelt 2001: 18–23). This is not simply because those who manage the machinery of the state want to increase its functions, but because it makes sense in light of a long-standing commitment by governments to defend public health.

Box 6.1   Nurses and health promotion

Nurses are expected increasingly to play an important part in health promotion. This might include participating in health education, screening procedures and campaigns to reduce health inequalities (see Gott and O'Brien

1990). District nurses, for example, are actively engaged in attempts to reduce health inequalities by working with people who are housebound and
those unable to access primary health care facilities. They also work to provide health education to help people manage their own chronic conditions
(see Nursing in Practice 2006). It should be appreciated that in order to
work effectively in health promotion, it is often necessary to be politically
aware and active in the community. Rather than concentrate solely upon
the medical problems facing a patient, nurses and other health care professionals have to address many of the economic, social and environmental
problems facing the communities in which they work (see Whitehead 2003).
It has been pointed out, however, that nurses often face a number of obstacles from within the health system. In a survey of five primary care trusts on
Merseyside, it was found that nurses often lacked suitable administrative support and had to challenge obstructive views held by many colleagues. Many
of these views related to out-of-date notions about what a nurse should do
(see Winters et al. 2007).

Theoretical perspectives

Why does the state provide health care? Is it to cure us of sickness or to improve
our levels of health? Those who believe in the former might wish to argue that
the state has no business in health promotion and that health promotion in
some way poses a threat to the freedom of the individual. Should the state tell
us what we can and cannot smoke, drink or eat? Should access to state health
care be limited to those who look after their own health or is it something that
we all have a social right to? We should be aware when discussing health promotion strategies that state involvement in health promotion is contentious.
It could indeed be seen as being far too intrusive.

Arguments for health promotion

Health promotion can be defended as an attempt to reduce the costs of providing state health care by intervening in the lives of individuals before their
health needs become too acute. Rather than rely primarily upon treating the
sick, early intervention could help to prevent illness and therefore relieve pressure upon the scarce resources marshalled by state-funded health care systems.
It has been argued that if we concentrate upon fulfilling needs, then greater attention should be placed upon health promotion and preventative measures.
If successful, preventative measures could reduce our need for expensive services. This applies in particular to the care offered in hospitals (see Sheaf 1996).
We could foresee a situation where primary care does far more than respond

to the immediate health problems of patients and dedicates a greater amount of time and resources to health promotion.

Enhancing freedom
Health promotion could be viewed as something that enhances our freedom by helping to guide people to a better understanding of their own best interests. It could be argued that the state has an important role in helping us to overcome the numerous barriers to real freedom. From this point of view, the state can help individuals strive for and in some cases reach their potential by improving the general levels of health, education and security of the community. The state could thus be used to provide what is best for people (see Taylor 1979). By empowering health professionals to intervene in the lives of individuals, they could have a beneficial impact upon the lives of individuals and communities by encouraging people to embrace healthy lifestyles.

Cross-party support
One of the most startling features of the case made in support of health promotion is that its supporters are drawn from across the political spectrum. In Britain, health promotion has been supported by key figures in the Conservative Party, the Labour Party, the Liberal Democrats and the Greens. Take a look at the following:

- *Conservative*: The Conservative Party (1987) claimed that the NHS must be more than a mere sickness service and that resources should be placed into promoting good health and preventing illness. Virginia Bottomley, the Conservative Minister of Health in 1994, claimed that the NHS must look beyond treating illness and concern itself with promoting good health. For example, people should be encouraged to eat healthy diets. She was careful to point out, however, that this did not mean that the NHS should refuse to treat those who failed to look after themselves and who have ailments that could be viewed as self-inflicted (Bottomley 1994).
- *Labour*: In 1992, the Labour Party identified a number of important measures to promote the nation's health including a complete ban of tobacco advertising, enforcing tighter regulations on the labelling of food, increasing the provision of occupational health services and restoring free eye sight tests. It claimed that increasing the amount of time that GPs have with their patients is one of the key measures needed in promoting health (Labour Party 1992). The Labour government pledged its support for health promotion but soon found that its resolve was being challenged by vested interests. In the early stages of the Labour administration of 1997 onwards, the Department

of Health targeted smoking and the advertising of tobacco products. The government buckled, however, following aggressive lobbying by sports that relied upon sponsorship from the tobacco industry (North 2001). This led to delays in the banning of advertising tobacco products.

- *Liberal Democrat*: The Liberal/SDP Alliance (the forerunner of the Liberal Democrat Party) was in favour of increasing investment in primary care, preventative medicine and health education programmes (Liberal/SDP Alliance 1983). The Liberal/SDP Alliance (1987) claimed that more should be done to improve primary care and health education. This was seen to be an essential step to transform the NHS and to focus at least some of its energies towards heath promotion rather than simply treating illness. The Alliance argued that the government should ban tobacco advertising, increase vigilance over food labelling and commit resources to tackling the problems of alcohol abuse and smoking. The Liberal Democrats argued subsequently that more resources need to be put into health promotion and that the NHS concentrates too much upon combating illness rather than encouraging people to take more responsibility for their own health. It was argued that this increase in role for state health care could be funded by increases in taxation on tobacco, which could also help reduce the incidence of smoking-related illness (Wallace 1997: 94–7).

- *Greens*: Greens have argued that many of the ailments we suffer from in modern society (including cancer and cardiovascular conditions) are products of the way we live, work and interact with our environment. The medical profession is criticized for failing to give due weight to these environmental factors and for treating the symptoms rather than the causes of poor health. According to many Greens, it is important that we look for ways to improve and sustain good health by improving our diets and by taking greater responsibility for our own health. It has been argued that the NHS in Britain is guilty of allowing people to take too little responsibility for their own state of health by providing paternalistic care for people who are taken ill. In their view, it makes more sense to increase resources for health promotion and discourage people from assuming that the health system will always be there to patch them up.
  (Gorz 1980: 149–50; Porritt 1984; Green Party 2000)

As we can see from the above, the main political parties in Britain are agreed that the NHS should promote health, provide health education and preventative services and encourage people to live healthy lifestyles. This is good news for the long-term development of health promotion strategies in Britain.

Scenario 12   Example of a traditional health promotion approach

Mandy is a 13-year-old girl, whose parents describe her as 'slightly chubby'. She is not keen on sports and likes to play at home on her computer. Her mother sometimes worries about her and often gives her chocolate and sweets to cheer her up. The school nurse has noticed Mandy's increasing weight and has spoken to Mandy giving her information to take home and a healthy eating plan.

Questions

1   To what extent do you feel the school nurse is giving Mandy the right advice?
2   Should more be done to assist Mandy?
3   Do you believe that health care professionals should provide unsolicited advice on weight issues? If so, why?

Arguments against health promotion

By concentrating upon what we should do, those involved in health promotion might face resistance from different sections of the community. Wall and Owen (1999) point out that the middle classes in particular are reasonably aware of healthy options but might refuse to change their behaviour because these options do not necessarily fit well alongside other pressures in their lives (Wall and Owen 1999: 142). For example, there are benefits to be had from going for a run or attending a gym but these activities might have to be slipped in alongside a demanding career and domestic responsibilities. Although a person might be aware of the importance of taking exercise, finding enough time could add to existing stress levels. Such barriers to living a healthy lifestyle might not count as an argument against health promotion in itself but it surely casts doubt upon the possible effectiveness of programmes to improve health. How many times do we hear 'I would love to be fitter but I just don't have the time' or 'I would love to eat healthier but there is so little choice in the canteen'? These limitations are real and their impact upon levels of health should not be underestimated.

Threats to freedom

It could be argued that health promotion, especially when this means providing unsolicited advice and attempting to control individual behaviour, can be a threat to the freedom of the individual. Arguments could be constructed to defend the freedom of the individual to consume the recreational drugs of their choice. If limits are to be placed upon these individuals, it could be argued that such limits would only be legitimate if it could be proved that the freedom of these individuals damaged the freedom of others. Even if we did not want to take the argument this far, a convincing case could be constructed against the state intervening in health promotion. Sheaf (1996) argues that by attempting to create a culture to influence behaviour, health promotion is a form of social control and health promoters should be criticized for attempting to impose their own values on the general public. Health promotion or preventative care can increase the blaming of victims. It can extend the jurisdiction of medical officers over the lives of the population and lead to increased demand (at least in the short run) for health resources (Sheaf 1996: 87). Individualists will often value the maintaining of control over our own minds and bodies and argue that we should be vigilant in defending our personal space and lifestyle choices against an intrusive, unrepresentative and potentially malevolent state. Apart from anything else, those forms of health promotion that target and monitor individuals could be viewed as yet another method of surveillance and control used by the state at the expense of the individual. Those who view life in these terms will undoubtedly be critical of health promotion and want to limit as far as possible the intrusions of the state into our private lives.

Conflict with other values

Health promotion campaigns can sometimes conflict with other value systems. Religious sensibilities, in particular, might stand in the way of certain health promotion activities. In the United States, for example, needle exchange schemes for intravenous drug users have been prohibited in some of the states and in Britain the government has refused to make sex education compulsory in schools (Roberts et al. 2001: 128). Religious groups in Britain were also actively hostile towards the safe-sex campaigns promoted by the government. AIDS was seen by some religious groups as a 'self inflicted scourge' and some took advantage of AIDS to condemn homosexuality and to assert the virtues of chastity. Fitzpatrick and Milligan pointed out that the response of some sections of the church resembled the 'social purity' movement of the early twentieth century in its attitude towards venereal disease. The state was called upon to discourage promiscuity rather than provide advice on safe sex (Fitzpatrick and Milligan 1987: 44). Although good health is generally regarded in a positive way, poor health stemming from what some regard as 'deviant' behaviour tends to reinforce the convictions of those who hold puritan values and make some people considerably less sympathetic towards the plight of others.

Scenario 13 An example of an anti-health promotion approach

Let us return to Mandy and to issues around her weight. The school nurse has noticed Mandy's increasing weight but feels that it is the parents' responsibility and therefore does not intervene except to monitor her weight. She does not want to intrude on family life by giving unwelcome advice.

Questions

1 To what extent do you think that parents should be concerned about Mandy's weight and address the problem?
2 Should the school nurse do more to help? If so, what could be done?

The third way

A third way approach to health promotion can be seen in the Labour Party's policy document *Choosing Health: Making Healthier Choices Easier* (DH 2004). John Reid, the architect of this document, claimed in the preface that the debate on health promotion has often focussed on the polar extremes of state responsibility versus individual responsibility. The state could, for example, intervene to limit individual choice by imposing constraints and by banning actions that pose a threat to our health. Alternatively, health could be left to 'whatever the hidden hand of the market and freedom of choice produces' (DH 2004a: 5). Here are the two main approaches, which have been referred to in this book as social democratic and neo-liberal. The first relies upon the state, the other upon the individual.

But there is a third way. Reid believed governments should be in the business of promoting health. He claimed that health promotion should focus upon changing people's behaviour and that this relies upon building support among people. All the government can do is provide guidance and opportunities and help to 'create the conditions' within which people can make healthier choices (Reid 2004a: 2). Reid believes that the government has an obligation to empower individuals to change their own behaviour and to support individuals in the choices they make (Reid 2004b). Rather than coerce people or simply leave them to fend for themselves, the third way involves calling upon the government to support and assist individuals and empower us all to become more independent of state services. The third way approach casts the state in the role of facilitator and reminds individuals that they have certain responsibilities in society that include taking more control over their own lives, health and welfare. This approach asks people to be realistic about their needs and to make use of the assistance offered by the state. The third way recognizes that health promotion can be used to empower individuals, enhance their freedom and, in the long run, make them less dependent upon the health service and upon services provided by the state. Rather than see health promotion as an intrusion, its benefits for both the individual and the community are highlighted.

Scenario 14   The third way approach

Let us use again the case of Mandy to illustrate a different approach to health promotion. In this version, the school nurse has noticed Mandy's increasing weight and has invited Mandy and her parents to some after school 'cook and eat' sessions so that they can learn to cook healthy meals together. Based on the family's interests, she has also suggested some local countryside walks and bike trails where the family can go out and have fun.

Questions

1 How realistic and useful is this approach to health promotion?
2 To what degree does this approach empower the family to promote their own health?

Policy developments

There is a long history of governments legislating to influence the lifestyle of citizens and to promote health. For example, attempts have been made by public authorities to control smoking since the seventeenth century. King James 1 increased taxes on tobacco in 1616 and smokers were punished in Russia, China and in the Ottoman Empire. In Russia, for example, smokers were mutilated and those who sold tobacco products were flogged to death. Although the British government has been aware since the 1950s of the causal link between smoking and lung cancer, it has been reluctant until recently to intervene; partly because it relies so heavily upon the revenue from taxing tobacco products (see Baggott 2000). Policies to restrict smoking in public places can be viewed as an infringement upon individual freedom or as a necessary step to advance the common welfare. Some of these policy developments will be included in what follows.

Britain

Although it is always possible that governments could be motivated by philanthropic concerns, it is often the case that governments intervene in social affairs because of dire need. In Britain, the government turned in earnest to health promotion campaigns following the problems it had recruiting for the Boer War in the early years of the twentieth century. When it had to turn down 40 per cent of recruits on health grounds, the government began to take health care seriously. This led to the creation of new services (including hospital care) for pregnant women and to the development of hospitals to deal with infectious diseases (Fatchett 1994: 62–3). Given its significance for all citizens, the authors suggest that health promotion should have a central role in the public provision of health care and should not be viewed as an optional bolt-on. We should remember that one of the original aims of the NHS was to promote health and well-being rather than simply provide medical care to the unwell. It was not, however, until the 1970s (in response to escalating demands upon the health service) that the government began to look again and take seriously the pledge to improve the health of the nation. From the mid-1970s onwards, Labour and Conservative governments have stated that more resources need to be diverted towards health promotion (see Fatchett 1994: 64, 82; Wall and Owen 1999: 137). Governments have recognized that state health care is expensive and that public demands upon the NHS are close to insatiable. Frightened of escalating taxation and further crises in the funding of welfare services, many governments are looking for ways to reduce our expectations and urge us to be more responsible for our own well-being. Rather than provide more health care to more people, we are encouraged to live in healthier ways. As governments attempt to place limits upon the direct public provision of health care, it would appear that health promotion attains increasing significance.

Health promotion provides an important way to tackle problems of poor health. For those actively involved in health promotion, a health service that ignores preventative measures creates real long-term problems for itself. According to the Health Development Agency in Britain, assisting people to adopt healthy lifestyles is often cost-effective. The Health Development Agency has pointed to the relative success of anti-smoking campaigns and those campaigns designed to promote safe sex; both of which targeted young people (Health Development Agency 2004: 1–2). It is recognized, however, that individual and collective action is necessary for health promotion to be effective. In a House of Commons (2001) report on health, it was noted that individuals are often insufficiently engaged in improving their own health and the health of the community. Although it was recognized that it is very difficult to influence people simply by telling them that their behaviour might pose serious risks to their health, it was considered important to find ways to encourage people to take responsibility for their own well-being. This does not mean that it is all down to individual effort. The Department of Health has argued that there should be a collective sense of responsibility for public health and that it is important to involve individuals and community groups in combating health problems. The Department of Health acknowledges that the government should be responsible for providing services to treat the sick and that it should also help to protect health by minimizing the social, environmental and behavioural factors that can damage the health of both the individual and the community (DH 2001a: 5–8, 21, 42–3). The Labour government under Gordon Brown renewed the Labour commitment to preventative health care and claimed that the NHS had an important part to play in helping people to improve their health and their life chances (DH 2008d). It would appear that health promotion is not simply a service that people can choose to consume or ignore. Social and political agendas are set regardless of personal indifference and it is these agendas that might be seen to threaten or enhance individual freedom.

Choosing health

Choosing Health (DH 2004a) is one of the most important landmarks in the development of health promotion in Britain. This rather lengthy policy document grew out of extensive consultations conducted between April and June 2004 with community groups, the general public, health care providers and the business community who were asked to express their views on a range of public health issues. People were asked to consider what the government should do to promote health and what should be left to individuals (DH 2004a: 12). In many ways, the Labour government was deliberately looking for an alternative to excessive state intervention on the one hand and individualism on the other. This, it should be remembered, is at the very core of the third way.

The consultation exercise for *Choosing Health* found that people accept they have responsibilities for their own health and that an overwhelming 88 per cent of respondents said that they were opposed to the government telling them how they must live. It was deduced from this that people want to be free to make choices about how they live and do not want decisions made for them. The government could assist not by dictating how somebody must live but by providing reliable information and support to people once they have decided to change their behaviour. This does not mean, however, that health professionals need to be passive in their dealings with patients. For example, health professionals were asked to consider the long-term benefits of health promotion 'even when advice on giving up smoking, exercising or changing diet is unwelcome and may initially make relationships difficult' (DH 2004a: 128). It was argued in *Choosing Health* that the government can not leave it to individuals to reform themselves and that it needs to cooperate with others to 'provide collective support to help to create an environment which promotes health' (DH 2004a: 6). It was found that many people expect the government to help create the right conditions and provide suitable support if and when they are ready to make a change to the way they live (DH 2004a). It is clear that the public want the government to limit its intervention so as to pay due respect to the sovereignty and personal identity of the individual.

Although the Labour government recognized the importance of giving people freedom to choose the way they live, it was also noted that the choices we make can sometimes have a negative impact upon others and that it is important to strike a balance between 'allowing people to decide their own actions, while not allowing those actions to unduly inconvenience or damage the health of others' (DH 2004a: 6). *Choosing Health* states that there is widespread support for the government to intervene where the choices made by some can have a detrimental effect upon the health of others and that the government needs to find ways to 'prevent people from doing things that put the health of others at risk' (DH 2004a: 15). The Labour government therefore sought to place limits upon smoking in enclosed public spaces in the belief that the actions of smokers posed a threat to the health of those who shared their space.

To those who would argue that this constitutes a dangerous extension of state power and jurisdiction, the Labour government justifies its policies on the grounds that it is seeking to empower people. Partly in order to avoid the accusation that central government is interfering too much in the life of the individual, the Labour government emphasizes that local community groups should have a key role in health promotion. Instead of depending upon central government, Labour policy calls upon voluntary and community groups to play an active role. It is felt indeed that these decentralized groups are closer to the patient and are capable of facilitating and coordinating collective effort (DH 2004a: 79–95). It is important moreover to recognize that the Department of Health wants to see patients developing their own personal health plans with some guidance from on-line resources and from personal health trainers drawn from and working within the patient's own community. This is regarded as a movement away from 'advice from on high to support from next door' (DH 2004a: 103). It is believed that such measures can help individuals gain more control over their own health and enable people to transform themselves according to their own interests and on their own terms (DH 2004a). According to the Labour government, this shows how state activity can nourish and strengthen individuals rather than make them subject to state power.

Smoking

Based in part on the foundations laid in *Choosing Health*, the British government introduced a ban on smoking in public places in July 2007. The smoking ban in Britain was designed to cover enclosed public places but exemptions are allowed for hotels, private members clubs, prisons, care homes, oil rigs and specialist tobacco shops (DH 2004a: 99; DH 2007a: 18). Before the ban was introduced, the Department of Health (DH 2004a) acknowledged that this was a sensitive issue because it involves a debate and conflict between our rights as individuals and our responsibilities to the community. According to the Department of Health (2002b), a smoking ban should help to reduce deaths and illnesses from smoking-related diseases, help people to give up smoking, improve air quality and improve the quality of life for people at work and at leisure. Research shows that a smoke-free environment in leisure facilities does not have a detrimental effect upon the leisure industry and improves the productivity of their workers. In California, for example, the respiratory health of bartenders has improved considerably as a result of a smoking ban in bars (see DH 2002b). Smoking bans have also been shown to have a beneficial impact upon working environments. These benefits include improvements in the health of workers, the reduction of claims for compensation made by employees against their employers and reductions in both fires and cleaning costs (DH 2002b: 20). The smoking ban is backed by a series of penalties, which can be enforced by the local council. Employers have responsibility to ensure that the smoking ban is observed and can be fined heavily if they fail to enforce the ban. These penalties far outweigh those imposed on individuals who smoke in a no-smoking area (Scottish Executive 2005; DH 2007b). While this might seem quite severe, the legislation has been introduced not to punish smokers but to promote the health of the community. The point is missed if we see this as a conflict between smokers and non-smokers. It would appear that the legislation seeks to improve the air quality of enclosed common spaces for the benefit of all.

The United States

The federal government in the United States is reluctant to play a major role in health promotion. This might be because of the individualist political culture. It would not be politically expedient for the American government to be seen to prescribe to its citizens what they should eat and how they should live their lives. This does not mean that the federal government has no role. Federal government has coordinated health promotion and health education since the early 1970s, but community groups (often with the backing of charitable foundations) are considerably more active in health promotion (see Lincoln and Nutbeam 2006). The Healthy People Programme, for example, relies upon extensive community action by citizen groups. These groups have coordinated their efforts, with a little help from the United States Department of Health, to tackle health inequalities and to empower individuals to make informed decisions about health issues. This project has found that individuals and groups are willing to work with each other on issues that directly affect their own lives (United States Department of Health 2001). Rather than run the risk of appearing too intrusive, federal governments in the United States leave the bulk of health promotion work to citizens themselves.

Smoking

The federal government in the United States has raised awareness of the dangers of smoking. Smoking has been banned on all domestic flights within the United States since 1987 and the US Environmental Protection Agency has run a number of campaigns on the dangers of smoking (Fitzpatrick 2001). Although there is no federal ban on smoking in public places in the United States, legislation has been introduced in the majority of the component states. In California, for example, people are not allowed to smoke in an enclosed workplace (Californian Department of Industrial Relations 1995). The level of fines for non-compliance increases with each successive breach of the law. There is generally a high level of compliance and respect for the law against smoking in enclosed public spaces. This has been attributed to the extensive educational campaign waged in California against smoking and the dangers of second hand smoke (Californian Department of Health Services 2001). In New York, a smoking ban applies to places of work, bars, restaurants, public transport, educational establishments, hospitals and childcare facilities (Department of Health: New York State 2003). Prior to the introduction of the ban, it was feared that restaurants would lose up to a quarter of their business. This does not appear to have happened. According to New York City Health (2007), restaurant profits have increased, new restaurants have opened and the health of those who work in restaurants and bars has improved considerably.

International examples

Many countries have embraced health promotion, especially since the 1970s. The World Health Organisation has been particularly important in showing that although lifestyle choices do have an impact upon our health, these choices are made within the context of our economic, social and environmental circumstances. It has been recognized that concentrating purely upon the lifestyle of individuals can lead to people being blamed for their own poor health rather than helped to make improvements (O'Connor-Fleming and Parker 2001). But different political cultures require different approaches. While some approaches to health promotion target the individual, others seek to draw in the community (see Blank and Burau 2004). These diverse approaches seem to reflect broader political differences between societies.

Health promotion strategies that target the individual often attempt to convince people of the benefits of living a healthy lifestyle. Approaching health promotion in this way is consistent with those societies based upon individualist values and where individuals are viewed as being primarily responsible for their own health and health care, such as in the United States and in Singapore (see Blank and Burau 2004). This approach lends itself to health promotion campaigns in which people are depicted as owning their own health like any other asset and benefiting from adopting healthy habits.

The alternative approach rests upon targeting the community. According to Blank and Burau (2004), this is a distinguishing feature of health promotion strategies in New Zealand and Sweden. In New Zealand, for example, health promotion is tied up with campaigns to reduce health inequalities. Rather than focus upon the individual, it is thought that improvements in health need to be pursued through collective efforts (see Blank and Burau 2004). The power of communal action can also be seen clearly in the approach taken in Sweden towards placing restrictions on smoking. Instead of simply trying to convince individuals that smoking is bad for them, the Swedish government has introduced bans on tobacco advertising and placed restrictions on where people can smoke. In an attempt to encourage healthier lifestyles, the Swedish government had increased investment in parks and placed restrictions upon traffic in residential areas. Rather than impose such policies from above, the government has involved local residents groups in the planning process (see Allin et al. 2004). Similar community involvement takes place in Australia where health promotion is approached by concentrating upon building healthy communities and by encouraging people to work together to improve general levels of health. The community focus in Australia is considered particularly important in multicultural work, especially in reaching people in the aboriginal community. Women's groups and environmental groups have been at the forefront of health campaigns in Australia and seem to have benefited from the support available via the state (O'Connor-Fleming and Parker 2001; Strategic Inter-Governmental Nutrition Alliance of the National Public Health Partnership 2000–2010 2001). By concentrating upon health in the community, health promotion campaigns can gain a great deal from the energy and enthusiasm of community activists. Making use of the voluntary sector can also help the state avoid being seen to interfere too much in the lives of its citizens.

Conclusion

We should remember that there are many types of health promotion and that while some types of health promotion might be intrusive other types would be seen by many people as helpful at best and harmless at the very least. A poster campaign encouraging us to eat more fruit and vegetables is unlikely to offend even the most stubborn and committed of meat eaters. Although many types of health education could be regarded as benevolent, attempts to place restrictions upon the behaviour of the individual may well encounter resistance from a sceptical public. Health messages can be viewed as attempts by the governing class to impose their tastes on other sections of society. If this is the case, governments and their health agencies could be viewed as petty tyrants and as potential threats to individual freedom. The solution to some of these problems would seem to lie in the way that health promotion is carried out. There is a major difference between being told what to do by the government and state health care and being provided with suitable support if we decide we want to adopt healthy lifestyles. Voluntary sector groups can help build bridges into communities. Although charitable foundations could fund these groups, this would not necessarily lend itself to a coherent health promotion strategy. The state must surely have a role in health promotion, even if some of the front-line work is carried out by organizations outside of the statutory sector.

7 Rationing

Chapter Contents

The term rationing may well conjure up images of wartime deprivation, queues and hardship. For people who lived through the Second World War and its immediate aftermath, the thought that services offered by the British NHS have to be rationed must hurt. When the NHS was formed, it promised to care for the citizens of England and Wales throughout their lives regardless of their ability to pay for medical treatment. But health care has become increasingly expensive and, in an attempt to place some kind of limits upon the budget of the health service, the NHS has found itself reducing what it has to offer. In this chapter we discuss and help try to answer the following questions:

- If health care is to be rationed, how should this take place?
- Should some procedures be excluded from the health care on offer by the state or even under health insurance schemes?
- Should resources be used to care for some categories of people (for example, the young) and exclude other categories (for example, the elderly)?
- Should people in work be given preference over those out of work?
- Should smokers be offered the same level of treatment as those who do not smoke?
- Should intravenous drug users or alcoholics be denied treatment for conditions stemming from their own particular addictions?

- If any of the above is denied treatment, what are the social costs and consequences?

The very notion of state health care systems rationing health care is controversial partly because any acceptance that rationing should take place will involve us in placing limits upon the extent of care on offer or the rights of certain groups of people.

Rationing

According to the Department of Health in Britain, rationing should be seen as a way to ensure a fairer distribution of services rather than a crude instrument to cut costs. It is suggested that rationing should be applied in particular to non-urgent treatments (DH 2007). There is, of course, a major problem here. What is urgent for one person is not necessarily urgent for another. How can we possibly measure the impact of a condition upon the life of another? For example, should counselling services be provided free of charge to people suffering from depression? The impact of depression upon an individual's life and the lives of their friends and family can be dramatic. We will certainly come across a number of these ethical dilemmas as we proceed through this chapter. For now it is worth taking note that some form of rationing is present in the vast majority of state health care systems. Despite its aims, commentators have pointed out that there has always been some form of rationing in the NHS. Busfield (2000) pointed to the existence of rationing by:

- delay – through the use of waiting lists;
- exclusion – by restricting access to specialists;
- age – as a result of preference being given to the young.

It is also worth taking note that during the 1980s and 1990s many countries formalized the ways in which health care resources were rationed. These countries included the United States and Norway (1987), Holland and New Zealand (1992), Finland (1994), France and Sweden (1995) (see Dean 1996). As we will see, there are many ways to ration services. These include placing a limit upon the services available and by increasing investment in one area at the expense of another. The latter method is known as priority setting.

Priority setting

Priority setting could be seen as rationing with a positive message. Instead of leaving us feeling as if something has been taken away, priority setting can appear to be a positive thing. The logic is as follows: there are limited resources, we need to make sure that these resources reach those who are most in need, we need to set priorities. Priority setting can be regarded as the process by which we determine the distribution of resources for one thing compared with another (see Busfield 2000). For example, the resources used to establish and run premature baby units could be diverted in part into health promotion schemes or outreach work to monitor and enhance the physical and psychological health of new mothers (Busfield 2000: 150–1). In choosing between options, we set priorities and ration resources. Consider the distinction between chronic and acute services. Resources are often concentrated in acute services where there is an immediate need and where delay in receiving treatment can be life threatening to the patient. This will leave fewer resources for the treatment of chronic conditions, despite the long-term pain and suffering of those who suffer from chronic illnesses (see Busfield 2000). This is a form of priority setting and perhaps one that few people would object to. If your local hospital had to close either its accident and emergency department or its stroke rehabilitation unit, what would you choose? Apart from anything else, a hospital without an accident and emergency department may well appear incomplete to local residents.

Theoretical perspectives

The idea of needs can be useful as a foundation to discuss rationing and the allocation of resources. A distinction can be made between economic and social models of need. The economic model of need concentrates upon the efficient allocation of resources and emphasizes the importance of securing the maximum benefit to the patient for the minimum cost. Priorities are thus set in the allocation of resources and prudence is encouraged in the decision-making process. The social model of need takes a more holistic approach and gives greater credence to the values and opinions of patients, which are considered primary in the priorities set (Fatchett 1998). The choice would therefore seem to be quite clear. Should we adopt a business-like approach and consider various demands upon health resources from an economic point of view or should we see these demands in their social context and make decisions based upon the needs of the patient? As we shall see, those who argue in favour of rationing often resort to using an economic model of need whereas the argument against rationing often embraces a social model of need.

Arguments for rationing

Arguments in support of rationing often proceed from either economic or therapeutic foundations. State health care systems might not have the resources to provide all that we want but might, with some creative decision makers, be able to respond to our more pressing needs. Those who support placing limits upon what the NHS does are keen to point out that individuals can and should take out private insurance to gain access to a broader array of procedures (see Pike 1991). Arguments can also be made for rationing on the grounds that not all procedures are of benefit to the patient. It has been argued that some procedures in obstetrics cause more harm than good (see Parker and Suzman 1995). For some of those who argue in support of rationing, the decision on what to ration should be made at a strategic level and not left to evolve in a chaotic and inconsistent fashion. Palmer (1996) claimed that governments must take tough decisions on rationing and not leave these decisions to those who administer the health service. Indeed, resources could be released by reducing the amount spent on administrators. This has been supported by senior academics in health care. Sir Roy Calne, Professor of surgery at Cambridge University, has argued that rationing is inevitable as the costs of modern medicine and surgery outstrip the resources available. He saw rationing as the only fair way to distribute resources. He criticized the increase in bureaucracy in the NHS and argued that patients are discharged early, wards are shut and there are too few beds partly because attempts to reform health care are often resisted by the vested interests of doctors (see Fletcher 1996). According to this line of thought, rationing is necessary to protect state health care from the pressures of unrealistic expectations and soaring costs.

Using the economic model of need

The economic model of needs is a rather blunt instrument. This is recognized by at least some of those who argue in support of rationing. According to Busfield (2000), simple calculations based upon supply and demand do not apply well when dealing with the allocation of health resources. Attempting to balance supply and demand fails to take into account the origins, intensity and severity of health needs and neglects to address the difference between what we need and what we want. It also tends to assume that clinical work or intervention is good in itself when it should be evident that this form of intervention may not always be appropriate. For Busfield, the NHS should refuse to finance some treatments and look into developing low cost solutions to health problems. She argues against the right of women to choose to have a caesarean for their own comfort and convenience and believes that the health benefits of elective caesareans are too small to warrant the high costs. The argument put forward by Busfield can be applied to lots of other areas. Why should a state health service respond to the wants of patients? Is it not more important that the needs of all citizens are prioritized?

The benefits of economic formulae

Health economists are keen to develop formulas to determine how resources should be distributed. One such formula, the Quality Adjusted Life Year

(QALY), attempts to measure the likely impact of a medical intervention upon patients' quality of life and the number of years they are likely to benefit from such an intervention. The impact upon quality of life could be measured by taking into account such things as the mobility and levels of distress experienced by a particular patient (Busfield 2000). The advantage of this method is that it provides an impersonal formula that can be used to consider the merits of different demands upon services. This formula takes into account the likely benefits of a procedure, both in terms of its effectiveness and the length of time a patient will benefit. Using this formula, corrective surgery for a child would usually score higher than many treatments for an elderly patient. This could of course contribute towards problems of ageism in the allocation of resources.

The importance of transparency

If some form of rationing or priority setting is used in state health care systems, do residents, taxpayers and citizens need to be made aware of the limits placed upon the service or the priorities set for funding health care? Malcolm Dean (1996) argues that an open system of rationing would allow for a greater degree of accountability to the public and it would allow the public and patient groups to challenge decisions made by those who ration resources. Commentators and policy makers have suggested that the existence of rationing is not necessarily a problem as long as overt criteria are used in setting priorities (see Appleby 1992), the decision-making process is open to scrutiny (Jones 1993) and 'fixed rules' are used in the allocation of resources (National Health Committee 2004: 2). So what might this involve? Overt criteria and 'fixed rules' could specify on what grounds a service is withheld, reduced or prioritized. If a service is to be cut, is it because it is too expensive, it benefits too few people, it is ineffective or of questionable medical value, or because resources are needed for more important procedures or services? We need to be aware, however, that what is important is by no means self-evident and that value judgements are necessarily made in fixing the criteria for rationing.

Scenario 15   Demonstrating the need for rationing

Pauline is 48 years old. She is quite overweight but not classed as morbidly obese, weighing 17 stone. She has tried for many years to lose weight but there are always lots of cakes where she works and she has a sweet tooth. She works on the top floor of her building but always takes the lift. Sometimes her weight gets her down and she has read in a magazine about gastric band surgery and has been to see her GP. He has discovered that the local NHS will not pay for her treatment as it currently in debt and might have to close one of their specialist children's wards.

Questions

1 To what extent should state health care pay for Pauline to receive this treatment?

2 What other measures could she take to reduce her weight?

Arguments against rationing

The case against rationing will often take into account social factors ignored by many of those who support rationing. If we are driven primarily by economic considerations, it is possible to view state health care in a fairly cold way. Those in control of budgets might ask 'what can we get for our money?'. This question could be asked without any regard for the social circumstances of patients. The poor are often hurt more from rationing because they are generally less able to afford private health care. Restricting access to abortions, for example, could have a disastrous effect upon the lives of those who are already experiencing hardship (see Brindle 1991; Pilkington 1995). Failure to take into account the circumstances of patients can create further problems for those who are already struggling and compound further the problems of health inequalities.

Ageism

Rationing procedures often hit the most vulnerable sections of the community. Evidence suggests that elderly people are often discriminated against in the allocation of health care. During the 1990s, it was estimated that approximately 20 per cent of coronary care departments discriminated against elderly patients who needed emergency heart treatments and there were reports of elderly patients being refused life-saving drugs (Fletcher 1994). Rationing health care can, indeed, contribute towards ageism in health care. The older we get the more health problems we are likely to face and the more expensive we become to state health care services. Viewed economically, the elderly might seem like a drain on the system. Viewed socially, they are citizens with rights to access services without discrimination. Elderly people might have more complicated health problems but this should not make them a burden.

Needs

Arguments against rationing ascribe more importance to responding to the needs of the patient than to dealing primarily with the costs of treatment. There might be circumstances that lead us to question whether the resources of state health care should be spent on those who jeopardize their own health. If our health problems are self-inflicted, then should we expect treatment to be there when we need it? If we follow this line of argument, we might be inclined to start constructing lists of self-inflicted ailments that do not warrant treatment under state health care. This list might include illnesses stemming from smoking, alcohol or drug use, over-eating, lack of exercise, participating in dangerous sports, unprotected sex and so on. However, if we concentrate upon responding to health care needs it makes no difference how these needs arose. Self-inflicted illnesses would thus be treated in the same way as all other illnesses. Sheaf (1996) reminds us that self-injury or non-compliance are 'failures of rationality on the patient's part, not evidence of an absence of need' (Sheaf 1996: 83). Although health care professionals might be judgemental about certain types of ailment, this should not impact upon the care they provide.

Public perspectives

Rationing is not popular among the public, especially in Britain. Polls conducted in the 1990s showed that public opinion was critical of rationing, even if that meant that taxes would have to increase to pay for improvements in service. Members of the public, however, were also shown to be critical of providing expensive treatments for those whose ailments were self-imposed through such things as smoking or alcohol abuse (Timmins 1995). McRae (1994) claimed that the public is becoming less deferential towards health professionals and less tolerant of rationing procedures in the NHS. This was attributed to a heightened awareness among the public of their rights as patients and was manifest in the belief that their rights were being attacked through the use of informal rationing procedures. Such evidence illustrates the strength of public support for a well-funded state health care system in Britain.

Box 7.1   Health care professionals on the problems of rationing

Health professionals understand the social costs of rationing as a result of their contact with patients. Nurses have argued that rationing health care can be a false economy because illnesses can progress and become more acute and expensive to treat. Health care workers can often find themselves in a difficult position when services are denied. This applies, in particular, within the NHS where patients feel that they are being denied their entitlement to health care. Nurses have also found themselves facing dilemmas when they are told to discharge patients from hospital early in the interests of cutting costs and making beds available. This is thought to conflict with their training and professional commitment to providing suitable levels of care (see Wells 1995). For health care professionals, rationing health care might be in the short-term interests of the health service but it can clearly create other problems and result in increased drains upon health care provision.

Scenario 16   Demonstrating arguments against rationing

Think back to our scenario involving Pauline and the problems she has controlling her weight. Having been denied surgery, she has gained a further 2 stone and now weighs 19 stone. She has now developed type 2 diabetes and needs further medical support. The GP argues her case with the local NHS and it is agreed she can have gastric band surgery.

Questions

1   To what extent has rationing health care created further problems for Pauline?
2   Should Pauline now have access to gastric band surgery through state health care?

Policy developments

Policy developments on rationing tend to be more covert than initiatives to tackle inequalities or promote good health. Few policy makers would see rationing in a positive light. If anything, it could be viewed as a sign of failure to provide a comprehensive service. Rationing often takes place in an informal way. Rather than being something to celebrate, it might be cast as a regrettable necessity. Consider the fortunes of a political party that openly advocates the use of rationing compared with one that promises to maintain a comprehensive system of state health care. Which of these parties would receive the more favourable treatment in the media and in public debates? If we expect the state to provide an extensive system of health care, rationing is difficult to justify. As we will see, however, rationing techniques are applied in a variety of ways in many countries.

Britain

Rationing is located at different levels and stages of state health care provision. Klein (1993) identified five different layers of rationing or priority setting in Britain. Rationing was said to take place through:

- fluctuations in the level of funding given to the NHS;
- the distribution of funds between regions and services;
- the priority given to different treatments;
- determining who should receive treatment;
- determining how much to spend on each patient.

It is apparent that Klein's list starts at the governmental level and works down the level of resources available to each patient. This is useful to illustrate that rationing does not simply take place at the level of patients competing for resources but is anchored upon decisions made at the strategic or budgetary level. A different approach to rationing can be seen in the ways in which Light (1997) identified some limitations in the NHS, which resulted in rationing through:

- delay because of waiting lists;
- under-staffing of health care professionals;
- under-investment in facilities;
- limited service, especially in the range of tests on offer.

Approached in this way, rationing could be seen to be the inevitable outcome of prolonged periods of under-investment rather than the result of a deliberate rationing strategy. Under these conditions, health administrators would have to make difficult decisions about how scarce resources can be distributed.

Building a comprehensive service

It should be apparent from what has been covered already that the notion of rationing sits uneasily alongside the original ethos of the NHS. The Labour governments of 1945–1951 set up the NHS in the belief that all citizens had a right to decent health care regardless of their ability to pay. It was assumed that there would be a heavy demand for the service in the early years but that this demand would reduce once the nation's most serious health needs had been attended to (see Fatchett 1998). Both Labour and Conservative governments for much of the post-war period remained committed to funding the NHS to deal with the most pressing needs for health care. It is clear, however, that resources were always limited and governments were soon forced to consider setting priorities for the NHS. By the early 1960s, both the Conservative government and the Labour opposition recognized the need for reform in the NHS. Rudolf Klein characterizes the period 1960–1975 as the 'politics of technocratic change' in the health service. He claimed that 'the debate was about instruments rather than ideologies, about means rather than ends' (Klein 2001: 49). Klein believes the NHS created new demands for health care and that there would never be enough resources to satisfy these demands. Because of this, the NHS evolved during the 1950s 'from an instrument for meeting needs (as conceived by the founding fathers) to becoming an institutional device for rationing scarce resources' (Klein 2001: 31). Attention was thus given to finding ways to make the NHS more streamlined and efficient while maintaining a broad commitment to providing a high quality service.

Rationing and the internal market

The Conservative governments of 1979–1997 showed a particular interest in making the NHS more business-like and indeed placed limits upon what the NHS offers. One way of doing this involved introducing an internal market through which health care providers competed with each other for business. Although this increased the amount spent on administering the health service and created further inequalities in access to health care, it was welcomed by some health care professionals (most notably by public health directors) as a useful tool to allocate resources (see Baggott 1998: 196–202). The internal market effectively made it plain that transactions take place in the NHS within relatively clear economic boundaries. The various branches of the health service knew how much money they had and needed and how this translated into the costs of treatment. Health professionals (and health administrators in particular) were thus involved in a series of commercial transactions, where budgets were split between different types of care and priorities were set in what might appear to be a cold business-like fashion.

New Labour and evidence based practice

While the internal market sits easily alongside neo-liberal approaches to health care and with the economic model of need, the cold logic of the internal market runs counter to the softer strains of New Labour and its philosophy of the third way. As we have seen, New Labour and the third way place more emphasis upon tackling social exclusion and upon active state involvement in setting agendas for the health of the nation. It seemed, at least in the early years of the Labour government, that rationing health care had no place in the philosophy of the third way and in the practice of New Labour. But the Labour government inherited the same problems of a vast health care budget and seemingly unending demands upon the health service. Rationing or priority setting was thus introduced, this time in the form of evidence based medicine or evidence based practice.

Evidence based medicine or practice involves setting guidelines for clinical interventions. Clinical trials are conducted to provide evidence of what is effective and what is not. This evidence is then used to produce guidelines on best practice. In consultation with health professionals, patients and various stakeholders in the community, coordinating bodies like the National Institute for Clinical Excellence (NICE) and the National Technology Board (in Scotland) help to identify those procedures that should be given support by the state health care system (see National Health Committee 2004; NHS Scotland 2008). Although these organizations aim to promote high standards and improve the experience of patients (NHS Scotland 2008), their recommendations can be seen as a way to place limits upon what is offered under state health care and can thus be viewed as a form of rationing. This is sometimes to the annoyance of medical professionals (see Box 7.2).

***

Box 7.2   Health care professionals on the problems of evidence based practice

Conflicts can arise between the recommendations of NICE and the judgement of medics. According to Benbow (2007), a consultant psychiatrist, the reluctance of NICE to endorse the use of drugs to retard the progress of Alzheimer's is in conflict with the General Medical Council's guidance which states that doctors must not withhold treatments deemed to be in the best interests of the patient. Benbow claims that most medics believe that it is in the best interests of the patient to slow the development of Alzheimer's by providing appropriate drugs. We should remember, however, that this is a value judgement. It could be argued, indeed, that slowing the development of Alzheimer's can prolong discomfort for the patient as they become increasingly aware of the condition developing.

***

The United States

The approach to rationing in the United States is rather different. As health care in the United States relies so heavily upon the private sector, access to health care is limited by a person's ability to pay for treatment or by the terms of their health insurance. State health care exists as a safety net for those who cannot afford adequate cover. It is not designed to provide a comprehensive service and is therefore less constrained by the high expectations of the public. Policy makers, however, have still wanted to find ways to limit what is provided by the state. One way of doing this involves excluding the range of treatments on offer. Public discussions held in 1994 in Oregon revealed that state funded health care was over-loaded and that cuts could be made by placing limits upon the number of treatments available through state health care. Through public debate, a list of priorities was created. This list was meant to be flexible and it was thought that the list would change during different stages of the economic cycle. Although the treatments available might shrink during periods of economic decline, it could expand during more prosperous times (see Guglielmo 2004). The Oregon experiment identified a minimum package of treatments that would be available in state health care facilities, but also excluded a variety of treatments including cosmetic surgery, sex changes, weight loss programmes and treatments for minor ailments like colds (Department of Human Services 2007). In this way, the public was involved in rationing its own health service. By asking people to prioritize the services available, policy makers hoped to create a greater consensus and popular support for the limitations implemented.

Relying upon state health care is not really an option in the United States. We should note, however, that rationing also takes place in the private sector where rationing could be seen as a method used to protect vested interests. In those health services that rely heavily upon private insurance and managed care plans, rationing techniques could indeed serve the interests of insurance companies. Critics have argued that the health care system in the United States is far too bureaucratic and that it fails to respond to social need and to listen to patients (Loewy 1999). According to Woodward (2001) the health system in the United States is constrained by financial and bureaucratic interests and managerial techniques are used to limit the treatment available in the interests of those who finance health care. The moral of the story is clear. Having health insurance does not guarantee access to all the health care needed. Health insurers will place limits upon what is available to their clients and the profits of these insurers will rely upon excluding certain treatments and on limiting how much individuals can draw from their insurance policies.

International comparisons

The sections on rationing in Britain and the United States reveal two distinct ways to approach rationing. Although the outcome might be the same and there is undoubtedly some cross over between the approaches, the priorities in the two countries are rather different. In Britain, the emphasis seems to be on assessing the benefit of certain procedures. This assessment can take place for each particular patient or be prescribed by NICE guidelines. In America, the favoured method involves excluding certain treatments. Both approaches are used in a variety of countries.

The severity of condition and benefits of a procedure
Services can be rationed according to whether they are deemed to be necessary and beneficial. This often involves considering the severity of a condition. Norway was the first country to introduce explicit rationing techniques in 1987. It was decided very early on that rationing should be based upon severity of condition and the possible consequences of denying treatment (National Health Committee 2004). In New Zealand, this approach has been adapted and used in developing the following criteria for receiving treatment:

- the severity of condition;
- the effectiveness of treatment;
- the impact of a particular condition upon the ability to work;
- the role of a patient in caring for dependents.

(see DH 2007)

In New Zealand, policy makers have deliberately rejected excluding particular treatments as a way to ration resources. The preferred alternative involves developing guidelines to help define when an intervention is considered sufficiently beneficial (Feek et al. 1999). Decisions at a strategic level about the scope and direction of the health service in New Zealand are not taken solely by politicians or even medics. Policy makers have involved a variety of stakeholders including health professionals, patient groups and the general public. This is thought to 'enhance awareness of the issues and constraints that surround decision making, and thus make them more accepting of prioritisation outcomes or more willing to address the factors that create these constraints' (National Health Committee 2004: 3). Clearly, there will always be some controversy over what is severe and what is sufficiently beneficial to warrant the spending of public money.

Excluding treatments

The other popular alternative relies upon excluding treatments from a list of services available. Rationing policies in the Netherlands attach importance to increasing investment in technology and standardizing the protocols used in medical decision making. A list of services that would receive public funding has been created, which ranks treatments according to whether they are necessary and effective. An attempt is made in this way to judge to what extent both the individual and the community benefits from medical interventions in a particular area (National Health Committee 2004). Rationing has been introduced in Sweden because of the severe strains that exist upon its state health service. These strains have arisen in part because of an increase in the number of elderly patients, children and political refugees in Sweden (Bergmark 2000). Although there is universal access to health care, some limitations have been placed upon placed upon the treatments available. Members of the public are said to expect a fairly comprehensive service given the high rate of taxation they pay, but some services are excluded in such areas as cosmetic surgery, IVF and the correction of bat ears (see Holm et al. 1999). In Sweden, the Parliamentary Priorities Commission was established in 1992 to develop principles and guidelines to be used in deciding where the priorities for health care should lie. A hierarchy of principles was created consisting of:

- equality of human dignity;
- treating the most needy;
- cost efficiency.

It has been noted that the third of these principles (cost efficiency) is considered less important than human dignity and treating the needy. This could be seen as an illustration of the importance of social justice in Sweden (National Health Committee 2004). It shows, moreover, that rationing health care does not need to rest upon purely economic factors and that other social factors can be considered.

Conclusion

Although the economic model of needs recognizes the importance of responding to the needs of the patient, it considers these needs in an economic context. The reality of fixed budgets places a limit upon what can be done by state health care and if the economic model of needs is employed it is possible to justify rationing by making use of the impersonal language of business. We should recognize, however, that if rationing procedures are to be applied it is important that the criteria for allocating resources is known. State health care is not free. Citizens pay for their health service through either taxes or some form of social insurance. In return for this payment, or as a result of possessing social rights stemming from citizenship, people will expect to be able to access treatment when needed. By what criteria, if any, should this treatment be denied? It is evident that the various stakeholders in state health care find it hard to agree. Managers are understandably driven by economic criteria. Medics have to use their judgement about clinical effectiveness. But what about social need? It could be argued that a patient who does not have the money for private health care has a greater social need for treatment than one who is fortunate enough to have money to spend on alternative health cover. This social need should be taken into account by state health care systems as they have no other way of securing suitable treatment. The approaches taken in both New Zealand and Sweden show that this can be done.

PART 3
PATIENTS AND HEALTH PROFESSIONALS

8   Patients' rights

Chapter Contents

We now turn to the issue of assessing the balance between the rights of patients and those of health care professionals. We should at the outset remind ourselves that the health system exists for the sake of patients rather than for health care workers. Just as academics are sometimes guilty of believing that universities exist for their convenience rather than for their students, health professionals might sometimes have similar attitudes towards their patients. Regardless of any career aspirations, it should be clear that without students or patients there would be no careers to develop in universities or health systems respectively. Health professionals must be aware of, and interested in, the needs of patients. Patients are not passive, compliant, obedient and clueless. People are now better informed about health matters and are better able to make choices for themselves than previously. Many people self-medicate to relieve minor symptoms. They use the internet to research their conditions and to find a suitable treatment. Some people use alternative therapies (like herbalism or homoeopathy) rather than rely upon conventional health care. Patients are indeed situated in a mixed economy of care. For many patients, before they visit a doctor they will decide whether the visit is necessary and what they hope to gain from it. Do they want medication? Do they want a referral to hospital or to some specialist treatment? It would be wrong to assume that all patients enter a doctor's waiting room in a confused state, unable to understand what is happening to them and desperate for any treatment or care. It seems more likely that many patients have a reasonable knowledge of the problems they face and have definite expectations of health care workers. In this chapter we consider and discuss possible ways to answer the following questions:

- How much credence should be given to the views of patients?
- What kind of rights should patients have?
- Should patients be viewed as autonomous?
- Should the relationship between health professionals and their patients be based upon an equal partnership or should ultimate power reside with health care workers?

The power and influence of patients is increasing. Part of this could be attributed to policy developments in different countries, but it undoubtedly flows in part from a cultural shift in health care systems. Goodyear-Smith and Buetow (2001) argue that there has been a move in medical circles away from a paternalistic approach to one that is firmly centred on the needs of the patient. Prior to this, doctors in particular have been cast as exploiters who have failed to give due weight to the opinions and expertise of their patients. They have been criticized for treating adult patients like children rather than as adults who have considerable understanding of their own bodies, lifestyle and values. People have become increasingly mistrustful of doctors and this has manifested itself in calls for doctors to have restraints imposed upon them. It has been argued, moreover, that in this atmosphere of mistrust it has become more difficult for doctors to help their patients (Goodyear-Smith and Buetow 2001: 450–2). As we will see, one response to this problem has been to call for the rights of patients to be extended. Has this gone too far or not far enough?

Theoretical perspectives

When looking at the arguments for and against the rights of patients it is worth remembering that extending the rights of patients does not have to be at the expense of health care professionals. There is not a finite pool of rights that need to be shared out. If we view health care workers and their patients like two opposing armies, each with their own interests and unable to negotiate, then it be will difficult to find ways to strike a balance between these two groups. On the other hand, if we view the relationship between these two groups as a partnership that is subject to change and revision we might be in a better position to understand at least some of the rights and obligations of each group.

Arguments for patient rights

Extending the rights of patients could make it considerably easier for health workers to do their job. On an individual basis, patients who are aware of their conditions and their needs for health care could be a lot easier to treat with than those who are unable or unwilling to articulate their needs. Patients can also provide health systems with important information about the needs of patients, the successes of the health service and where gaps in provision exist. The Department of Health in Britain recognizes the importance of consulting patients and patients' groups and claims that this can help to provide reliable information about the needs of patients and of the community. Understanding what the community wants in terms of health care can also assist health professionals to make improvements to the service they provide (DH 2008b). If we attempt to deny patients their voice, health care workers will be left having to guess what patients need and the health service will almost certainly suffer as a result.

Understanding the patient perspective

It is important that health professionals have some understanding of the patient perspective. This can help workers in health care to adapt their practice to the diverse needs of their patients and perhaps even identify some areas to explore in their own professional development. In an important document compiled for the Department of Health, Christine Farrell identifies some of the main reasons why involving patients in the development of health policy is so beneficial. She claims that gaining the perspectives of patients 'illuminates the patient experience and helps to shape a health service that is truly responsive to individual and community needs' (Farrell 2004: 4). These perspectives can be identified at various stages in the process of consultation. Doctors and other health care professionals can gain the insights of individual patients when treating them and of the broader outlook of patients in consultative committees. Patients can have an important role in these committees. In particular, they can provide new perspectives on the problems faced by the NHS as they are often not hampered by loyalty to any particular party. Members of the public who get involved in consultative bodies are thought to be motivated by democracy, altruism and community service though it is acknowledged that these people might be unrepresentative of the wider public (Farrell 2004). We will take a more detailed look at these consultative bodies later in the chapter.

Benefits to the patient

Patients can also benefit greatly from taking a more active role in the development of health care and in being more proactive in their own treatment. Farrell (2004) claims that patients respond favourably to being involved in shaping health provision and that this can contribute towards increased confidence, greater levels of understanding of issues among patients and better relations between patients and health care professionals. There are many ways to empower patients. These include spending more time on health education, involving patients in discussing their own treatment plans and involving patients in the development of services. It has been found that patients who feel in control of their own lives and are active participants in their own health care tend to have a greater chance of improved outcomes (Goodyear-Smith and Buetow 2001: 453). Farrell believes that patients should be treated as equal partners in the healing process and that enhancing the power of patients can increase the satisfaction of patients and lead to them having greater confidence in health professionals (Farrell 2004). According to the Department of Health (DH 2008d), giving patients better information and more choice about their health care has encouraged patients to assume greater levels of responsibility for their own health care and has helped to nurture a sense of partnership between health professionals and their patients. It would appear that an active and engaged patient is more likely to take positive steps to improve their own health than one who is passive.

The patient-centred approach to health care

The patient-centred approach to health care places value upon the views and experiences of patients. It is recognized that patient input is necessary to communicate effectively with medical practitioners and that failure to take into account the patient perspective can lead to non-cooperation and non-compliance with the healing process. Research conducted in the 1990s showed that patients rarely resist advice on physical problems and the need for antibiotics but that they are far more likely to resist doctors attempting to prescribe tranquillizers (Senior and Viveash 1998: 22). Holistic practice is one form of the patient-centred approach. By attempting to take into account the whole person holistic practice concentrates upon unravelling the complexities of the individual patient or client (Armstrong 1986: 45–8). Those who support the patient-centred approach to health care will recognize that services need to be designed around the needs of the patient rather than attempting to force the patient to fit existing services. This might mean, for example, supporting more people in their homes (DH 2006a: 4–5). It could be argued that all care should be negotiated with the patient. By working with individuals, families and communities, it should be possible to negotiate care with patients so that they feel more empowered and in control of their lives (Scottish Executive 2006a). A patient-centred approach to health care necessarily empowers patients. Instead of dealing solely with bio-medical conditions, practitioners are urged to deal with the patient as a whole and to find ways to engage the patient in the healing process (see Box 8.1).

Box 8.1 Health professionals' support for patient power

Many health care professionals are supportive of extending the rights of patients but this is often qualified by 'resistance to giving up their own control of the consultation' (Farrell 2004: 14). Patients are thus often treated 'instrumentally to achieve clinically preferred goals' (Farrell 2004: 14). Nurses have been shown to be particularly supportive of involving patients in the therapeutic process though 'their willingness to promote involvement can conflict with a professional ethic of protecting patients from negative and exploitative experiences' (Farrell 2004: 14). From this we can see that although some health professionals might want patients to be more involved in either the development of their own treatment plans or in influencing the running of services, the agenda is still firmly set by health professionals. This could leave some patients feeling that they only have a narrow sphere of influence.

Scenario 17 Illustration of the argument supporting patient power

Albert is a 57-year-old man who suffers from rheumatoid arthritis. He often gets flare-ups and finds that on some days it is difficult to carry out daily living tasks. Through Albert's GP he has just joined his local NHS's Expert Patient programme. This has enabled him to gain more knowledge and information about his condition and he has learnt what he can do himself to reduce the severity of his symptoms.

Questions

1 What do you think are the advantages and disadvantages of Expert Patient programmes?
2 What are the benefits to health professionals of empowering patients?

Arguments against patient power

Those who argue against patient power do so because they have a more traditional view of what it is to be a patient. All talk of empowerment, rights and choice might simply miss the point. It could be argued that patients visit their doctors and other health professionals to receive treatment and not to be cross-examined or negotiated with. According to Armstrong (1986), holistic approaches to health care can undermine patients by allowing health practitioners to probe ever deeper into the personal lives of their patients and by failing to give adequate attention to the social context of health. In tackling depression, for example, a holistic practitioner might look into the possibilities of using counselling rather than challenging the economic and social conditions that can give rise to depression (Armstrong 1986: 46). Arguments against extending the influence of patients can indeed be couched in the language of caring for patients and even protecting them from the realities of health care politics. Consider, for example, an elderly patient who needs a hip replacement. Would it benefit this person to know how much the procedure costs and what else could be bought with the money or would it simply worry them and make them feel guilty about consuming precious resources? The same could apply to patients participating in consultative groups. What insight can they have beyond their own personal experiences and how are these experiences going to be viewed by medics in the groups? The case against extending patient rights could point out that increasing the information available or making the system more transparent will not necessarily benefit the patient.

Lack of knowledge

Those who argue against patient rights often point out that most patients lack sufficient medical or scientific knowledge to make informed decisions about their own health care and patients should be willing to delegate responsibility to those who have sufficient knowledge. It follows from this that health care professionals are the better placed to make decisions on behalf of the patient because these professionals have been trained in or have access to medical knowledge (Tauber 2001: 311). Farrell claims that for many patients 'the limitations of personal knowledge about health problems or health care options compromise their ability to judge any decisions made about their health' (Farrell 2004: 13). Because they possess medical knowledge, health care professionals are thought to have an advantage over the majority of patients. Should health care professionals be in the business of educating their patients about their conditions or about the wider context of the health service or would this be an inappropriate use of resources? Is it more cost-effective to treat passive and compliant patients? If so, what are the consequences for patient rights?

Favouring the middle class

Increasing the scope for patients to make decisions about their health care or to influence the development of health services does not necessarily benefit a broad spectrum of society. Indeed, moves to increase the influence of patients might even increase inequalities in health care. Consider, for example, the assertion that the middle classes are generally better able to exert influence upon health care providers because of their educational background and their ability to communicate using a suitable and compatible language and style. If the patient voice is given credence, the middle classes could use their powers of persuasion to advance their own positions over and above those of other sections of society (see Dixon and Le Grand 2006). This argument recognizes that an active interest in health, health care and the health service is probably confined to relatively few people. While the middle classes might be happy to challenge and comment upon the service they receive, other social classes might have a far more instrumental view of the health service and view their own health and health care in a less proactive way. If this is the case, then is the call to extend the rights and influence of patients simply another device used by the middle classes to get their own way?

The problems with autonomy

Autonomy is something to be valued. It involves being free to make decisions to gain or retain some control over our own lives. But is our autonomy diminished when we are ill? Tauber (2001) argues that the principle of patient autonomy is misunderstood and valued too highly as an end in itself. In his view, the aim of medical intervention is to restore autonomy rather than respond to any supposed existing autonomy. He points out that in order to be autonomous, we must be capable of understanding our situation, be rational, be capable of moral sensibility and we need to be able to think of ourselves as being autonomous. When we are ill, however, we can lose sight of at least some of these abilities. Tauber is convinced that we need to recognize that (in the medical setting) we are often in a dependent position. He believes that people should be willing to be guided by experts and that autonomy is in reality 'an aspiration of the curing process, a goal, not a starting position' (Tauber 2001: 314. See also p. 300 and pp. 311–14). Both Tauber (2001) and Rothman (2001) believe that it is inappropriate to expect patients to behave as autonomous agents in a clinical setting because patients are often in a state of physical and/or psychological distress. This level of distress can often stand in the way of patients making informed decisions about the best course of action (see Rothman 2001: 257; Tauber 2001: 311). When patients are diagnosed with a serious and life-threatening illness, they might be interested in the options available but they would also benefit from the guidance of their health professional. To tell patients that it is up to them what they do would not be very helpful.

The obligations of patients

Critics of patient rights prefer to talk about the obligations of patients rather than their rights. According to Sorell (2001), patients have obligations toward the health system and other patients. Sorell believes that patients behave in a morally reprehensible manner when they cause harm to themselves, when they refuse to listen to and act upon the medical advice that they are given, when they fail to cooperate with doctors in their treatment and thereby waste the time of doctors and other health care professionals. Such actions are thought to deprive the health system of resources and divert attention away from other patients. In Sorell's view, granting autonomy to the patient can disrupt the relationship between doctors and patients and can only work if patients live up to their obligations and assume a share in responsibility for their own health and for the outcomes of medical intervention (Sorell 2001: 26–31). It could, of course, be argued that there are no rights without obligations. Concentrating on rights could be misleading by giving the impression that patients should have rights without any obligations on their part. It must surely be the case that the best interests of patients are not served by health professionals giving the patients what they want and ignoring what they need (see Box 8.2).

Box 8.2 GPs and the problems with patient autonomy

There is considerable variation among GPs in their respect for patient autonomy. It has been found, however, that GPs have a reasonable amount of respect for autonomy when patients are electing to try different complementary therapies. They are more reluctant to embrace patient autonomy on medical matters, especially if it challenges their professional judgement (see Rogers 2002). Daniel McQueen, a GP in Brighton, argued against patient power in a letter to the *British Medical Journal*. He claimed that to be effective it was important that doctors have knowledge of their patient but that patients cannot be equal in the relationship because they lack medical knowledge. He pointed out that patients may well have their demands satisfied by doctors but often at the expense of doctors denying their own skills (see McQueen 2002). GPs often find it difficult to empower patients, especially when this involves prolonged negotiation over treatment. According to Farrell, GPs 'see benefits predominantly in terms of compliance, management and control of a patient's health behaviour' (Farrell 2004: 18). Farrell notes that health professionals can be sceptical about patient power because patients often lack knowledge and they might be in a vulnerable state.

Scenario 18   Illustration of the arguments against patient power

Let us return to Albert who has joined an Expert Patients programme in the hope of finding ways to manage his rheumatoid arthritis. Through participating in the programme, Albert has learnt about a few new treatments which may slow down the progression of his condition. His GP believes he should remain on his existing treatment but Albert is adamant that he wishes to try a new treatment.

Questions

1   To what extent should Albert be able to request and demand new treatments for his condition?
2   What are the implications here for health professionals?

Policy developments

It might be the case that health policy has generally sought to promote the interests of patients but not necessarily their rights. As we have seen already, patients might want rights to things even if these things are not in their best interests. For example, somebody who is having trouble controlling their weight might want access to medication rather than change their eating habits and exercise routines. Here is an instance of a drug being used to deal with a symptom rather than the cause of a problem. Should patients have the right to choose their treatment and the drugs they are prescribed? It should be clear that when we talk about the rights and influence of patients, it makes more sense to concentrate upon the way that policies attempt to grant particular rights to patients (and perhaps even the responsibilities of patients) rather than to think in terms of the right of patients to get everything they want.

Britain

It took a while before the NHS in Britain turned towards giving patients a voice in their treatment and in the direction of the health service. The NHS was established and was run in a paternalistic way (see Forster and Gabe 2008). Patients were not expected to influence medical decisions. They were the recipients of treatment rather than the instigators of policy or medical practice. By the mid-1970s, however, gaining the perspective of patients was given value. Community Health Councils were formed in 1974 and continued to exist until 2003, when Patient Forums replaced them. The aim of these councils was to monitor health services on a local basis and to help patients if they needed to complain about the treatment they received (DH 2008b). It is apparent, however, that Community Health Councils were not very powerful. In the period 1979–1997, Conservative governments in Britain started to use extensive market research to elicit the views of patients rather than rely upon advice from Community Health Councils. Under these circumstances, Community Health Councils became marginalized and their members despondent (Forster and Gabe 2008). Fatchett (1994) argues that while in the early 1980s the NHS was driven by the needs and interests of employees, by the early 1990s it had been hijacked by the needs and interests of patients. Although this might appear to be empowering and democratic, the health service reforms of the Conservative government reduced the power of Community Health Councils, led to tighter control over the information given to the public and excluded the public from any real say in the way that health care was organized and delivered (Fatchett 1994: 48–51). Instead of involving patients in the development of health care, patients were granted certain rights under the Patient's Charter.

The Patient's Charter

The Patient's Charter was introduced by a Conservative government intent upon making health care and other public services responsive to the needs of those who use the services. This was a ploy in many ways to make the internal market appear to be less of a threat by attempting to convince people that they had certain rights as consumers of health care and other public services. Consumers of these services were informed of their rights and provided with information about the performance of the services. Efficiency targets were set, independent inspections carried out, and complaints procedures put into effect (for an account of the background see Kavanagh 1994). *The Patient's Charter* stated that it was important for the NHS to respond to the needs and views of patients, to establish clear standards and to acknowledge the rights of patients to access health care. These rights included the right to health care according to need, to be given accurate information, to have access to our own health records and to complain if the service failed to work in accordance with the standards set (see DH 1991). This approach is not always embraced by members of the health profession (see Box 8.3).

The Patient's Charter gave patients rights as consumers. It reiterated that British citizens have a right to health care and constructed a list of services that patients can expect. This has been criticized by some commentators. Renade argues that the *Patient's Charter* ignores that we have rights as citizens and 'the citizen is repackaged as a consumer and taxpayer, concerned with economic and market-based rights only' (Ranade 1997: 156). Fatchett likewise believes that too much is made of our rights as consumers and not enough of our rights as patients. She claims that even if we accept that patients are also consumers, the *Patient's Charter* does little to recognize the diversity of consumer interests in health. For Fatchett, the ethos of the *Patient's Charter* is far too consumerist (see Fatchett 1994). What these critics show is that patients are not merely consumers with rights. Any rights that patients have stem from something other than their purchasing power in the market. They ask us to consider what rights we have as citizens and where these rights come from. Do these rights stem from the payment of taxes or from being members of a society?

Box 8.3 Health care professionals and the *Patient's Charter*

The *Patient's Charter* was criticized by staff in the NHS because:

- it encouraged patients to expect a higher level of performance from the NHS without there being additional resources to guarantee improvements in service;

- clinicians argued that people should be treated according to need and not because they had been on the waiting list for a certain amount of time. Arranging procedures based upon the amount of time on a waiting list could lead to minor operations being given precedence over major operations (see Kent 1998).

Beneath this lies a broader problem. Patients' rights can be viewed as a list of entitlements granted to consumers of the health service that bears little or no relation to the ability of the service to cope with increased demand and pays too little attention to clinical judgement. For those who work in state health care, the formal declaration of patients' rights might be regarded as too one-sided and liable to inflate the expectations we have of state health care.

New Labour and patient rights

The Labour government of 1997 onwards subsequently overturned the provisions outlined in the *Patient's Charter* and replaced these with a broader commitment to involving patients in the development of the health service. The *NHS Plan* of 2000 (see DH 2000) contained measures to enhance the rights of patients including:

- improving communication between medics and patients by sending copies of relevant correspondence to patients;
- the development of patient surveys and forums;
- a system of patient advocates in hospitals.

Such measures show how the Department of Health wanted to find ways to collect the views of patients and to advance the rights of patients through providing them with help to deal with hospital bureaucracies. It should be noted that having rights as patients is not necessarily enough unless these rights are known to the patient and there is some help to guarantee that these rights are not violated. According to the Department of Health (see DH 2004b), the NHS is committed to consulting patients and involving patients at a variety of levels in the administrative structure. In particular, the Department of Health declared an interest in:

- what patients want from the NHS;
- how patient input can help to change attitudes in the NHS;
- extending choice to make the health service more responsive to the needs of patients;
- improving access to health care;
- reducing health inequalities.

The Department of Health has stated that it is important to listen to patients for only in this way will a responsive health service be created. Indeed, patients are no longer regarded as passive consumers of the health service but as active participants in the planning of state health care (see DH 2003b). This is a far cry from the original paternalistic approach of the NHS. The enhancement of patient rights can be seen in the ways in which patients can be drawn into managing their own health care and the scope given to patients to influence the development of health services in Britain.

Managing their own health care

When we talk about patients managing their own health care we need to recognize the importance of patient choice and the rise of the expert patient. The Labour government claims that it is committed to extending choice in the health service in the belief that choice is needed to meet 'the individual needs of an increasingly diverse population while also being underpinned by the values of fairness and equity we all hold in common' (DH 2003a: 6). In a survey conducted by the Department of Health, it was noted that patients want to be consulted about their treatment and that it is important that the NHS responds to 'the needs of each individual patient and recognizes their diversity' (DH 2003a: 56). One way of advancing the rights of patients in a therapeutic setting is through the Expert Patients Programme. Rather than see the patient as a passive recipient of care, Expert Patient Programmes look for ways to empower the patient through educating and involving them in the management of their condition. The Expert Patients Programme looks for ways to create partnerships between health care professionals and their patients and is used in particular in the management and monitoring of chronic conditions. An electronic health library has been created, a help-line for advice has been provided and guides for self-treatment at home have been produced. According to the Department of Health (DH 2001d), patients involved in these programmes become better equipped to deal with their conditions and need to visit health professionals far less frequently. Expert Patient Programmes are valued because they cut costs by making patients less dependent upon formal health care (see Forster and Gabe 2008). Because of this, these programmes could be seen as an alternative to rationing. Taking into account the awareness, interest and skills that some people have in matters concerning their own health, it makes sense to harness these abilities and in so doing attempt to reduce demands upon state health care. It is hoped that as a result patients will become empowered and the relationship between patients and health care professionals will be changed for the better. Rather than restricting their remit to the provision of health care, health care professionals become both educators and facilitators of health care.

Patients and the development of health services

Patients are involved in the development of health services in two main ways. First, there is the opportunity to participate in Patient and Public Involvement

Forums (see Opinion Leader Research 2005). These forums are involved in challenging poor service and in suggesting how improvements can be made. The forums involve patients, carers and families and are seen as providing a means through which local people can voice their views on health issues. Some members of Patient and Public Involvement Forums are cynical about how real the consultation process is. Research has shown that some of those involved in the forums believe that decisions have already been made before consultations begin and that the forums are nothing more than a token gesture. It is noted, moreover, that these forums tend to attract the usual suspects and rarely attract members whose first language is not English (DH 2005b).

Patients also get involved in shaping services through taking part in the Patient Advice and Liaison Services (PALS), which were set up to provide support and advice to patients and help them to resolve any problems that they might have with the health service. By monitoring the health service, it was hoped that the PALS system could advise the NHS about any notable gaps the delivery of services (DH 2009). The PALS system is sometimes criticized for being too complex and confusing for some patients and for being unrepresentative of the communities they serve (Baggott 2005). This is a recurring problem for community groups. These groups are often set up in the belief that governments are out of touch and in no way reflect diversity in society. Once established, however, many of these groups attract people who might see each other regularly in the committee meetings of different organizations. Taking part in the politics of a local community can be addictive and it tends to appeal to a minority of active citizens.

The United States

Whereas Britain has the beginnings of a well-developed sense of patient rights, this is rather less developed in the United States. As we have seen, the United States relies primarily upon a system of private health care. Under such a system, the rights of patients will be limited largely to what they can afford through their health care insurance packages. It is not as if patients' rights are not on the political radar. President Clinton was committed to developing a patient bill of rights but he was adamant that this should apply to all citizens of the United States. He talked about this in each of his annual addresses between 1998 and 2000 (White House 2000). Clinton was in favour of a bill of rights for patients that responded to the needs of patients and strengthened the relationship between patients and health care professionals. The bill was to include the rights to information, to participate in making decisions, to care without being discriminated against and would apply to private patients and to those covered by Medicare and Medicaid. Clinton also believed, however, that patients had responsibilities to maintain their own levels of health (see US Department of Health and Human Services 1999). This failed to attract sufficient support and a weaker bill, the McCain-Edwards-Kennedy Patient

Bill of Rights, was passed in the Senate. This applied to all citizens with their own health insurance and recognized the right of these people to choose their doctor and health care provider (see Democrats 2001). It is evident that where state health care is under-funded and insufficient to meet demand, the rights of patients will be less developed.

International comparisons

Formalized systems of patients' rights, either in the form of patient charters or a patient bill of rights, have been introduced in a variety of countries including Australia, New Zealand, Canada and Norway. Such initiatives have been designed to empower patients in their relations with health care providers (Government of Canada 2002). As we have seen already when discussing patient rights in Britain and the United States, there are at least two ways of approaching patient rights. The first is to see these rights as consumer rights. The second is to take into account the rights and responsibilities we have as citizens.

Consumer rights
It is often the case that the rights of patients are identified in documents similar in style to Britain's *Patient Charter*. In Australia, the *Public Patient's Hospital Charter* includes the right to receive free treatment in public hospitals and to use health care according to need rather than in accordance with the ability to pay (see Government of Canada 2002). There is also a *Private Patient's Hospital Charter* (see Australian Government Department of Health and Ageing 2007) in which the rights of private patients are spelt out in detail. These rights include the right to choose your doctor and to use services not covered by state health care such as physiotherapy, dentistry or optical work. Patients in Ireland have a number of rights recognized including the right to preventative health care, access, information, consent, choice, privacy and confidentiality, safety, personalized treatment as well as the rights to complain and to receive compensation for any harm caused by the health service (Irish Patients Association 2002). These types of rights are rights as consumers. They tend to identify a range of services available and thereby clarify the extent and limits of state health care. They do not in a real sense contain any expectations of the patient.

Rights and responsibilities in Canada
The alternative approach talks about rights and responsibilities and is framed not in the language and style of consumer rights but in terms of what citizens can expect and the responsibilities they have. This approach can be seen in Canada and has far more in common with the direction taken by Clinton in the United States and the Labour government in Britain. The Canadian

government recognized in 2002 that the views of patients had to be listened to because patients were becoming more knowledgeable and assertive about their needs (Government of Canada 2002). No doubt influenced by the spread of the internet and the cultural shift away from deference towards health care workers, patients are increasingly vocal about their rights. The New Brunswick Charter of Rights and Responsibilities includes the right to access public health care regardless of the ability to pay or the lifestyle of the patient. Health care is guaranteed on the basis of need. Within the same document, however, there is a section on responsibilities of patients to live a healthy lifestyle (Government of Canada 2002). This charter is clearly not one that concentrates solely upon the rights of patients. By stating formally that patients have responsibilities as well as rights, it inserts a measure of negotiation into the mix. The citizens of New Brunswick may well have the right to treatment according to need but they might also have to expect that health care professionals will remind them of their responsibilities. Here is an example of a charter that aims to identify some guidelines for the relationship between health care professionals and their patients rather than to list and quantify the rights of patients to health care (Government of Canada 2002).

Conclusion

Patients have rights. In some ways, it does not matter whether a government grants these rights to patients in a formal document or charter. We exercise our rights by participating in our own health care, by making decisions about what kind of health care we want or need and by challenging health care professionals when necessary. The old adage that 'doctor knows best' only applied when patients knew less about their conditions. Patients are increasingly able to make decisions and manage their own health. They have access to information (sometimes of dubious quality) through the internet and might even be referred to some of these sources in consultations with health care workers. This is not of course to say that health care professionals are no longer needed. It is more likely that the range of things that health care professionals are called upon to do is expanding. Health care workers play a vital role in our communities. They do not have to deal solely with our illnesses and our acute needs. They can help to keep us healthy and, in so doing, make us all less dependent upon state health care.

9   Professionalism

Chapter Contents

Health care professionals work within a complex web of power relations. As we saw in the previous chapter, the expectations that patients place upon those who work in health care are increasing. It should be recognized that patients have life histories, social circles, behaviour patterns, expectations and a multitude of social identities. Health care professionals need to be able to treat patients with respect regardless of their age, class, gender or ethnic background. Being aware that each of these will impact upon a patient's sense of self or identity should help those who work in health care to provide suitable treatment and advice. It is perhaps worth remembering that when a patient leaves the consulting room or health care facility, other parts of their identity take over. They are no longer patients and their priorities change. They return to their lives, their relationships, their communities and to a more familiar set of expectations.

In addition to responding to diversity among patients, health care professionals must also find ways to cooperate with colleagues holding different specialisms or performing different functions. Working in primary care, for example, involves a multitude of relationships. Health care professionals often work as part of a multidisciplinary team that could include doctors, nurses, pharmacists, health service managers, physiotherapists and so on. The number and variety of practitioners will vary according to the size and resources of a practice but it is clear that primary care offers many different types of service and expertise. Work in primary health care will also involve liaison with other statutory and voluntary agencies. Primary health care workers often find that at least part of their time is spent dealing with social services and with benefits agencies (Williams 2000). To work well in primary care, health care workers must be aware of what they can offer their patients and what needs to be provided by other people or agencies. This is sometimes known as sign posting.

In this chapter, we will take a look at a series of arguments about professional identity and ask to what extent health care professionals should have autonomy in their roles. This will involve taking a look at the outset at some of the arguments made for and against professional autonomy and then move on to consider how these debates relate to the working lives of doctors and nurses respectively and the challenges of working in a multidisciplinary team.

The nature of professionalism

The traditional idea of a profession rested upon the notion that professionals were people who had mastered their discipline and had gained expertise through individual effort and sacrifice. This view of the professions placed a heavy emphasis upon specialized training and upon having expertise in a particular area. The professional status of doctors, for example, derived from possessing such specialist knowledge (Wilkinson and Miers 1999; Gerrish et al. 2003; Wall and Owen 1999). This view of what it is to be a professional, however, is rather narrow. It tends to give the impression that anybody without a specialism cannot be regarded as a professional and that, in the context of health care, professional status and the power that goes with it should belong to an elite group of consultants and doctors. We should be aware that the power base in medicine has changed considerably since this idea was fashionable. New professions have emerged and have led to new (more inclusive) views of what it is to be a professional. Rather than emphasize the possession of specialist scientific knowledge, new views of professionalism place considerably more value upon reflective practice and upon multidisciplinary work. This tension between old professionalism and new professionalism will be explored in this chapter.

Theoretical perspectives

The theoretical perspectives on professionalism deal not so much with arguments for and against professionalism per se but with the arguments for and against traditional notions of professionalism. As we will see, those who argue against old professionalism are often trying to build a case in support of new professionalism.

Arguments for old professionalism

In this section on arguments for old professionalism, we will be concentrating upon the arguments made for the professional autonomy of doctors. According to Blank and Burau (2004: 22), professional autonomy is 'part of the implicit contract between doctors and the state'. They acknowledge that this relationship between doctors and the state does change over time. Sometimes doctors have freedom while at other times this freedom is curtailed (Blank and Burau 2004). This is not to say that doctors want freedom in all things but the freedom to make decisions about health care is considered paramount (see Fuller 1995). The professional autonomy of doctors is deemed to be important because of the following:

- Doctors have mastery over a complex body of knowledge that cannot be understood and regulated by amateurs (see Prechel and Gupman 1995).
- Possessing professional autonomy allows doctors to refuse to give treatments they consider to be useless or futile (Gampel 2006).
- Professional autonomy allows doctors to resist pressures from the political and commercial sectors (Emanuel et al. 2002).

For many doctors, professional autonomy lies at the very core of their sense of identity and is an indispensable feature of their vocation. Some have complained, however, that they have lost a great deal of their autonomy (see BMA 2005). Part of this could be traced to challenges mounted against old professionalism.

Arguments against old professionalism

Old notions of professionalism run the risk of breeding arrogance. Fuller (1995) argued that by assuming ownership over a specialist body of knowledge and by refusing to share this knowledge, doctors have created dependency among patients and a distance between doctors and patients (Fuller 1995). This distance has sometimes made it difficult for doctors to function well and to communicate effectively with their patients. Doctors are now called upon to develop new ways to view their relationship with patients and with other health professionals. Old notions of mastery (superiority stemming from specialist knowledge), autonomy (freedom from external control) and privilege (freedom from immunity) have been abandoned (see Royal College of Physicians 2005). Doctors, in short, have had to revise the way they view themselves and their relationships with others. Patients have increased their power, managers have increased their influence in running health care services and other health care professionals have increased their influence. Under these circumstances, it is no longer appropriate for doctors to assume superiority.

The case against professional autonomy

The notion of professional autonomy has been criticized for being too secretive, incompatible with accountability and hostile towards the rights of patients (Cannavina, Cannavina and Walsh 2000). As we have seen, the notion of professional autonomy was valued by doctors because it enabled them to follow their vocation free from outside interference. For critics of professional autonomy, however, it gives doctors a weapon to use against anybody who questions their judgement. This could apply to patients. Fuller (1995) argues that professional autonomy and old notions of professionalism stand in the way of doctors adapting to the needs of their patients and that this is increasingly inappropriate, especially in light of the diverse needs of modern communities (Fuller 1995). Professional autonomy can also serve as a barrier between doctors and other health care workers. Whitehead and Davis (2001) note that it can create significant obstacles to collaboration between health professionals in multidisciplinary teams. Doctors have been accused of being too domineering over other groups in the team and this applies in particular to professional relations between doctors and nurses. Critics, therefore, justify challenging professional autonomy on the grounds that it is necessary to shake doctors out of their remote and elitist perspectives on the world and remind them of their obligations to their patients and to their colleagues in multidisciplinary teams. It is apparent that these critics are less than charitable in their views towards doctors and that what they are describing does not reflect normal practice but abuses within the system.

The case for new professionalism

New professionalism is a considerably more democratic way to view the relationship between health professionals and their patients. Irvine (2001) notes that new professionalism moves away from the doctrine of autonomy and self-regulation and concentrates far more upon establishing partnerships between the public and health care professionals. According to Green (2006), contemporary views of professionalism challenge the defence of privilege and elevate the importance of sharing knowledge. New professionalism is based upon relationships, adapting to diverse needs and the importance of collective endeavour. Although it is hoped that this view of professionalism can be applied across the spectrum of health care, it is particularly suited to the ethos of contemporary nursing with its emphasis upon interpersonal skills, negotiation, communication and support, reflective practice and a more even distribution of power between nurses and their patients (see Wilkinson and Miers 1999: 32; Gerrish et al. 2003). Taken together, these values differ significantly from those advanced in old notions of professionalism. Rather than allow patients to be dominated by a minority in possession of scientific knowledge, new professionalism attributes greater weight to the cultivation of reflective practice in the interests of adapting to the diverse needs of patients.

Policy developments

This section on policy development will concentrate upon how the professions arrange themselves and work with other groups. Rather than concentrate upon government policies for different groups of workers, we will be asking how health care professionals relate to each other and to their patients. This will include examples from Britain and from other parts of the world.

Understanding power relations

There are two main theoretical frameworks that can be used to understand power relations. Pluralists argue that power is dispersed through a variety of groups participating in the health system. These groups cover the interests and express the views of administrators, health professionals, politicians and patients. Pluralists assume that there is no consistent bias in the balance of power between these groups. Each can exert influence (see Ham 1992). According to Annandale, the power base in contemporary health care should be seen in terms of 'a number of groups jockeying for position; as a game of move and countermove' (Annandale 1998: 235). This view of a multitude of groups vying for power is consistent with pluralism. It has been argued, however, that pluralists fail to take into account the power imbalance between health professionals and patients and that patients rarely exert effective influence over the organization of health services (Ham 1992). If pluralism is limited in its understanding of bias, what kind of alternative approaches can we use?

The main alternative is known as structuralism. Structuralists argue that there exists a definite hierarchy in the medical profession. At the peak are the medical practitioners. Corporate bosses (health planners and administrators) are seen as 'challenging interests' to the dominant power of the medical profession. Members of the community are seen as 'repressed interests'. Structuralists argue that the power of the medical profession rests upon its control over knowledge, training and in its professional autonomy. This is enhanced by the medical profession imposing its own concept of health, which is thought to emphasize the medical features (Ham 1992). As we have seen already, there are definitely moves to undermine this power base. Wider definitions of health that embrace social factors cut into the value of scientific knowledge. Patients and other health care professionals resist the hierarchy suggested by structuralists and draw our attention to the importance of seeing health care as a series of relationships that must be negotiated.

Changing boundaries

The boundaries between the various branches of health care are changing constantly. Reductions in the working hours of junior doctors have meant that nurses have learnt new skills and now perform more specialized tasks. Nurses are now being trained in universities rather than solely in hospitals. They have become key figures in health care and have helped to encourage a more holistic approach to health and health care. According to Annandale, the traditional distinction between nursing care and medical treatment is becoming blurred (Annandale 1998: 244). Take, for example, changes in regulations governing the prescribing of medication. Prescribing is no longer the sole domain of doctors. The Department of Health in Britain recommended in 1999 that the authority to prescribe medication should be extended to a broader range of health professionals including nurses, pharmacists and optometrists. It has been argued that nurses who have the authority to prescribe are able to work more holistically and this is said to improve relations between nurses and patients (see NHS Scotland 2003a; National Prescribing Centre 2004; Intute 2008). By taking on the role of prescriber, optometrists, pharmacists and nurses are helping to shift the balance of power within the medical system and advance the reputation of their own particular professions.

Doctors

The British Medical Association (BMA 2005) has argued that it is important to identify core professional values. It recognizes that the medical profession is steeped in ancient values (such as commitment, integrity, compassion and responsibility) and that these are still relevant today. It is felt, however, that doctors need to change with the times. The British Medical Association recognizes that as patients become better informed, the relationship between doctors and patients is being transformed and the way in which doctors view professionalism needs to adapt to the changing expectations held by patients (see BMA 2005). The power of doctors, however, depends a great deal upon broader social factors. Busfield (2000) noted that the power of doctors over their patients declines when doctors are directly dependent upon them for their income. In private practice, doctors tend to have a cautious and personal approach because their patients are often far more likely to question their judgement. Doctors have traditionally had more autonomy and power under the state system where patients (especially working-class patients) may well be less demanding (see Busfield 2000). The power relationships between doctors and patients are thus influenced considerably by the class system and by the confidence and economic power of their patients. It was noted in the previous chapter that middle-class patients in particular are adept at working the system and at challenging health care professionals. While this might be seen as a strength by those who feel able to hold medics accountable for their views and advice, it is clear that passive patients might still find themselves relatively powerless in their encounters with the medical profession.

The relationship between doctors and other health care professionals is also changing. Busfield (2000) notes that doctors have traditionally been at the top of the medical hierarchy in hospitals. Senior doctors grew to expect deference from more junior members of staff and nurses were expected to do more menial work. This pattern is, however, changing. New health care professionals, especially in the field of psychology, have avoided slipping into a subordinate role. Advanced nurse practitioners, who have specialisms and are able to prescribe medication, have also side-stepped the positions traditionally allocated to nurses. The logic of Busfield's argument seems clear. People who want to avoid working in subordinate positions in health care need to find ways to develop a specialism. This is one way of convincing doctors and others that they hold skills and insights that go beyond those necessary for routine work. In the context of multidisciplinary work, doctors still find that their position at the top of the hierarchy is questioned, challenged and overturned by managers and by other health care workers. According to the BMA (2005), there is no reason to believe that doctors should lead multidisciplinary teams. There is, indeed, a strong case to be made for equality among their members.

Nurses

Nursing has often been seen as lacking the characteristics of a profession, largely because nurses did not have the autonomy and power of self-regulation held by many professions. During the 1970s, nursing emerged as a distinct profession. Nurses in Britain began to work towards defining a knowledge base, which in time assisted nurses in their campaigns for greater levels of autonomy (Gerrish et al. 2003). Although it was felt that a university education would enhance the professional status of nurses and help to de-mystify medical knowledge, it has been found that many nursing studies courses take place in new universities and that nursing studies students are often isolated from students studying more traditional academic subjects (Maslin-Prothero and Masterson 1999). Studying at degree level, however, has been essential to augment the status of nurses among health professionals, to allow for the development of specialisms and for the development of new roles for nurses in the health service.

No longer seen as assistants, nurses have taken over many of the functions formerly performed by doctors. These functions include health promotion, consultations on minor acute illnesses and managing chronic illnesses. Nurses have in this way developed expertise in certain areas (see Wilson et al. 2002). Nurses have a particularly important role in primary care where they have a reasonable degree of autonomy. Practice nurses are often the first point of contact for the general public and their roles often include screening, primary prevention and administering immunizations. The majority of health promotion clinics are also run by nurses (see Ross and MacKenzie 1996: 157–8). This increase in responsibility, however, has created a number of problems. Nurses have been critical of increasing demands placed upon their time and of the assumption that they can perform a multitude of tasks. It has been argued that patients in particular have increased expectations of nurses and that this does not take into account the general lack of resources and overworking of staff in the British health system (Dillon 2001). Both the Royal College of Nursing and the trade unions have pointed out that nurses have to be more proactive in challenging under-staffing and poor working conditions. They have been urged, moreover, to attempt to influence the strategic development of the NHS (see Brindle 1997; Murray 1998). Many nurses, however, avoid political activity in the belief that politics is a 'deviant activity' that threatens to damage the 'caring ethic' (Maslin-Prothero and Masterson 1999: 218). Nurses therefore find themselves taking on a multitude of tasks and performing these tasks out of a sense of vocation and commitment to their patients.

It would appear that nurses face a dilemma. On the one hand, they are involved in trying to develop their own status as professionals. On the other, they are trying to empower their patients (Maslin-Prothero and Masterson, 1999: 223). As mentioned already, nurses might be required to spend less time with patients and develop specialist interests in order to enhance their own professional status. But this seems to undermine some of the dominant values held by nurses. It is worth bearing in mind that nurses might prefer to regard themselves as carers. It has been found that nursing students hold onto the view that nurses are first and foremost carers rather than independent health professionals (see Apesoa-Varano 2007). Even if this is the case, it is still important to recognize that nursing practice calls upon nurses to have a multitude of skills and abilities and that these can be used effectively to address the needs of patients. Caine et al. (2002) found that nursing-led care in a chest pain clinic was as effective as doctor-led care and that patients were more likely to take the medication recommended by nurses. Bradley and Nolan (2007) claim moreover that the development of advanced roles for nurses has great potential to improve services available to the patient, improve levels of cooperation between health professionals and lead to more debate and discussion about medicines and their effectiveness. The holistic and patient-centred approach taken by many nurses can indeed help to transform the health service.

But there are still barriers to the professional development of nurses. In particular, nurses seem to have had a long struggle to overcome resistance to their advancement from doctors. Maslin-Prothero and Masterson (1999) argue that the power relationship between doctors and nurses can be seen as a reflection of traditional patriarchal and class relations in society. They claim that the health system is skewed in the interests of men and that caring, something that is seen as a feminine virtue, is regarded as inferior to other medical skills. They note that doctors have more power in the relationship and that nurses often have to avoid openly challenging the power of doctors by relying upon making tactful suggestions. Even if doctors are open to nurses having more responsibilities, there are some concerns among doctors that transferring less complicated roles to nursing staff can mean that doctors are left to deal with more difficult cases. This does not necessarily reduce the workload of the doctor but simply makes it more stressful (Wilson et al. 2002). We should remember that when discussing the relationship between various health professionals, changes in these relationships can have a dramatic impact upon the workload of those who work in health care. If nurses take on the responsibility for running health promotion sessions, targeting health inequalities, community outreach work and running clinics, what is left for doctors may be considerably less interesting and rewarding. The kind of roles taken on by nurses allow for closer contact with patients and for making a real difference to the health and well-being of the people they see. Under these circumstances, the job satisfaction of nurses could well increase at the expense of doctors.

This shift in the functions and power of nurses within the health system is replicated in a number of other countries. Nurses have increased the range of tasks they have responsibility for in the United States and have made significant inroads into paediatrics, inner city clinics and in the field of occupational health (Asubonteng et al. 1995). In Canada, Advance Nurse Practitioners are able to diagnose disorders and prescribe medication (NP Canada 2007). In New Zealand, nurses are allowed to practise as independent prescribers. Although in practice they are often working alongside other health care professionals, they do have the authority to assess, diagnose and prescribe medication (Ministry of Health 2005). These developments do, of course, have their critics. Mollar and Begg (2005), for example, have argued that the rise of nurse prescribers threaten standards in health care because nurses are trained to provide care rather than to diagnose problems. They believe, moreover, that by taking on some of the roles of doctors nurses might undermine good team work, which relies upon each part of the team performing a distinct role rather than duplicating the tasks performed. For some critics at least the message is clear. Doctors and nurses have different levels of training and should stick to what they know best. If this were the case, it would place significant limits upon the professional development of nurses.

Scenario 19   Illustration of changing roles in health care

Gerry is an 85-year-old man with Coronary Heart Disease. He has been going to see the same GP for the last 40 years. He has tried to make an appointment with his GP but the receptionist has suggested an appointment with the practice nurse. Gerry insists on seeing his doctor as he has 'always looked after me'. Worried about Gerry, his GP makes a home visit to discuss his issues.

Questions

1 To what extent do you think that Gerry's GP is the only one who can give him the care he needs?
2 To what degree should patients be able to decide who treats them?

Conclusion

Patients' rights and professionalism do not have to conflict. If we hold onto an old view of professionalism, one based upon professional autonomy, then it is possible to see how there might be tensions between the rights of patients and those of health care professionals. But even this would only apply if professional autonomy were taken to mean that doctors need to be free to make and enforce their own clinical judgment. As we have seen, patients are often unwilling to be compliant and it would seem that the success of health care interventions rely to an extent upon giving due weight to the economic and social factors impacting upon the lives and values of their patients. Although old views of professionalism might conflict with the rights of patients, the same cannot be said about the new views of professionalism. New professionalism encourages practitioners to work in teams, to communicate with patients and to be reflective in practice. Applied to nursing, this could work well alongside a commitment to holistic treatment. New professionalism allows for patients to be viewed as active participants and contributors to the healing process. The suggestion here is that a balance can be struck between professionalism and the rights of patients but that this relies upon health care professionals adopting a holistic approach to health care.

10 Conclusion

Chapter Contents

The provision of health care

The distribution of resources

Patients and health care professionals

Conclusion

We have looked at a range of theoretical arguments and policy developments on a number of controversial issues. It has not been our intention to applaud or scapegoat any particular group or perspective, but to outline at least some of the possible approaches to issues affecting health care systems in different parts of the world. We have looked at policy developments in Britain, the United States and in a number of other countries including Canada, New Zealand and Australia. The aim has been to show how the state intervenes in these countries to shape the health care on offer to their citizens and to consider how these systems tackle inequalities in health, promote good health, ration scarce resources and deal with the potential conflicts between health care professionals and their patients. But can we go beyond this and use our knowledge of these theoretical perspectives and policy developments to engage in broader debates about how to organize health care?

This is certainly not the place to advocate a particular programme for health care. From what has been said already it should be clear that what is suitable for Britain will not necessarily suit any other country. Each nation has its own history of health care which would seem to reflect its dominant social and political values and the ideological convictions of particular governments. This does not mean, however, that what we learn from examining different theoretical perspectives and policy developments is not transferable. Each example we have included, whether these are theoretical or policy focussed, can be embraced or rejected and in the process help each of us to develop our own approach to health care. In particular, we could consider the options we have and the criteria we use to decide:

- Who should provide health care?
- What priorities should be set in the distribution of health care resources?
- How can the rights and responsibilities of health care professionals and patients be balanced?

In each case, we need to be aware of the options and that the issues addressed in these questions are related to each other. By approaching each in turn, we can start to develop a framework to understand a multitude of issues.

The provision of health care

In this book, we have looked at three main providers of health care: the state, the private sector and the voluntary sector. Some countries, like Britain and Sweden, have relied heavily upon state provision of health care since the Second World War. Others, like the United States, rely far more upon private health care. We have seen, however, that a mixed economy of care is becoming more common, particularly in those countries that have made extensive use of state health care. This mixed economy allows for care to be offered by a variety of providers.

But why should there by differences between countries in the way they organize health care? Many of the health systems referred to in this volume are based in reasonably prosperous countries. It could be argued that Britain, Sweden, the United States, Canada, Australia and many parts of the European Union could afford to provide state health care given the economic conditions in those countries. The reasons why countries differ in the amount they are willing to use the state no doubt has a great deal to do with differences in their political cultures. Countries like Sweden have a particularly well-developed sense of common endeavour and place a high value upon equality. For other countries, like the United States for example, freedom is more important than equality. This could mean that having the freedom to spend your own money is preferred to being taxed highly in the interests of promoting greater levels of equality. If you are to decide for yourself the extent to which the state should be involved in the provision of health care, you could begin by considering the relative importance of equality and freedom. The more you value equality, the more you are likely to want the state to intervene in the economy and to provide such things as health care, education, housing and so on. If on the other hand you wish to prioritize your own freedom, you will probably be less inclined to grant to the state such extensive powers and be far more supportive of private health care, private education and of individuals fending for themselves.

Discussions on who should provide health care can also be approached be taking note of the characteristics of the state and by considering to what extent the state is a suitable provider of health care. If the state is not suitable, then alternatives need to be identified. These alternatives could include the private sector or the voluntary sector. The state, it should be noted, is not always viewed as a benevolent institution. Placing our faith in the state could be foolish. Who controls the state? Who are the elites in the political system?

Can the state represent the interests of all classes, genders and ethnic groups? If not, whose interests are being advanced? If the modern state (especially in the countries included in this volume) is controlled by middle-class men, then what kind of policies can we expect from the state? If the state and the health, education and welfare services provided by the state are skewed in the interests of the minority, then what are the alternatives? Those with sufficient income may well prefer private provision, especially where state provision is either run down or struggling to keep up with demand. For those who are unable to afford such care, then the voluntary sector is undoubtedly important. This seems to apply in particular for people who feel alienated from the values promoted by the state. As we have seen, it often makes sense for voluntary sector groups to be involved in attempting to reach marginalized sections of the community who might regard the state with some suspicion.

The distribution of resources

How should resources be distributed? What kind of priorities should be set in state health care? If money is tight and health care resources are expensive, who should receive treatment? Should resources be distributed in favour of one group or another or should these resources be dedicated to certain types of service? Part 2 of this book addressed such thorny issues. We looked at the problems of health inequalities and asked to what extent the state should take it upon itself to reduce these inequalities. We also discussed health promotion and asked whether the state should be in the business of advising people how to live their lives. Finally, we addressed rationing health care and considered to what extent a fair system of rationing could be devised.

We venture to suggest that in a perfect world everybody would receive the health care they required. If the budget for health care was infinite, it might be tempting to believe that there would be no need to set priorities. Health care would be available according to need rather than according to the ability to pay. Health administrators would not have to choose between providing hip replacements for the elderly and running a premature baby unit. In those health care systems based upon private insurance, people would not have to fear the cancellation of their policies and being made dependent upon an under-funded system of state health care.

However tempting this might sound, there are still factors that harm the health of the individual that no amount of state funding could remove. When discussing health inequalities, we saw that some groups in society are suspicious towards the state and would prefer to access treatment from people in their own communities. Both the state and state health care can be viewed as intrusive and insensitive to the needs of different groups in the community. Health promotion programmes can be interpreted as the state attempting to force individuals to abandon their own culture and pastimes and adopt the lifestyle of other groups. We need to take this into account when discussing the politics of health care.

Let us not forget moreover that lifestyle is not the only factor influencing our health. There are many factors to take into account. Some will be genetic, others will be environmental. Some individuals will be predisposed to certain conditions as a result of their genetic makeup. Migraines, heart disease and a variety of other conditions run in families. Our social circumstances will also have a dramatic impact upon our health. It does not take a great deal of empathy to realize that people living in poverty and surrounded by crime will tend to live a more pressured and stressful life than somebody who is reasonably affluent and comfortable. The way we work also impacts upon our health. Do we work in dangerous conditions? Do we push ourselves in our careers until we have nothing more to give? If so, what damage do we do to our own health?

Even if we accept that priorities in health care need to be set, what criteria should we use? Should the aim of state health care be to tackle illness or promote health? Should marginalized sections of the community be given more resources to improve their health and well-being? It should be clear that those who value equality, social justice and community cohesion may well support such intervention by the state. Nothing could be further from the priorities of neo-liberals and those who believe that we should be responsible for our own health, health care, education, pensions and so on. According to this line of thought, the state should keep out of our lives and leave us to fend for ourselves.

Patients and health care professionals

In the final section of the book, we looked at the rights and responsibilities of health care professionals and patients and asked if these could be balanced. Although these chapters deal primarily with power relations between different groups of people, we need to remind ourselves that health professionals and patients are functioning within a world created for them by policy makers. Who provides health care and how priorities are set will influence how health professionals and patients view themselves and each other.

Let us consider this in a little more detail. If the state is the primary provider of health care, then citizens pay some sort of tax or social insurance to the state and will have expectations that the state will provide health care when they need it. Under a system of state health care, health professionals are public servants and patients might feel that they have certain rights to treatment. It could be argued, however, that patients have obligations or responsibilities to tend to their own health, to access the resources of state health care sparingly and to abide by the guidance provided by health care professionals. Patients do not necessarily have more rights under a system of state health care.

Under private care, the rights of patients are limited to what they can afford to purchase from health care providers. Private practitioners are not public servants but business men and women. They are not responsible for tending to the health needs of the nation, to reducing health inequalities or even promoting the long-term health and well-being of their patients. Private health care relies upon a series of commercial transactions. In a well-ordered system of private health care, patients will know what they are entitled to and health care professionals will know the extent and limits of their obligations to their patients.

For those who believe in a mixed economy of care, rights and obligations of both patients and health care professionals become even more important. In a mixed economy of care, the state, the private sector and the voluntary sector all offer services. Health care professionals can choose where to be based and will no doubt find that the expectations of patients vary greatly when accessing services from the different sectors. The rights of a patient when paying for private treatment will be rather different from those of patients using state health care or the voluntary sector. It could be the case, of course, that any particular individual has experience of all three simultaneously. State health care might be used to manage an illness. Voluntary sector groups might provide the individual with advice and activities to improve their health. Private health care might be used for specialist treatment of a particular condition. We should remember that the rights and responsibilities of both patients and health care professionals will be influenced by the ethos of the particular sector providing health care. The relationship between patients and health care professionals is therefore one subject to constant change and, in many ways, to a series of negotiations between both groups.

Conclusion

Rather than audit the nation's health, we have been engaged in a series of debates about health care. We have raised questions about the responsibilities of the state in health care and about the rights and responsibilities of patients and health care professionals. Although these debates have been designed to stand on their own, there are connections between the debates covered. We have outlined three key theoretical positions: the social democratic, neo-liberal and third way. These appear in a number of the chapters and can provide the reader with a theoretical thread upon which to hang the issues discussed. We have also looked at policy developments in a variety of countries. The book has used clearly defined sections so that readers who are interested primarily in policy developments in a particular country will be able to focus upon their area of interest. It is hoped that by including theoretical perspectives, policy developments, the experiences and opinions of health care professionals and by making use of scenarios, readers will be able to see health in its economic, social and political contexts and recognize that the health care we have (and might have in the future) depends to a large extent upon the values we embrace and promote as individuals and as a nation.

Black, D. (1980) *The Black Report*. The Department of Health and Social Security. www.sochealth.co.uk/history/black.htm (accessed 3 March 2008).

Black, M. and Mooney, G. (2002) Equity in health care from a communitarian standpoint, *Health Care Analysis*, 10: 193–208.

Blair, T. (2003) The third way: new politics for the new century, in A. Chadwick and R. Hefferman (eds) *The New Labour Reader*. Cambridge: Polity.

Blakemore, K. (1998) *Social Policy: An Introduction*. Buckingham: Open University Press.

Blank, R. and Burau, V. (2004) *Comparative Health Policy*. Basingstoke: Palgrave Macmillan.

Blaxter, M. (1990) *Health and Lifestyles*. London: Routledge.

Blendon, R., Schoen, C., Donelan, K. et al. (2001) Physicians' views on quality of care: a five-country comparison, *Health Affairs*, 20(3): 233–43.

BMA (British Medical Association) (2002) *Healthcare Funding Review*. www.bma.org. uk/ap.nsf/Content/healthcare+funding+review~healthcare+funding+review+ -+Mechanisms~healthcare+funding+review+mechanisms+-+charities (accessed 3 March 2008).

BMA (2005) *Professional Values*. Health Policy and Economic Research Unit. London. www.bma.org.uk/ap.nsf/content/profval (accessed 3 June 2008).

BMA (2007a) *Improved self care by people with long term conditions through self management education programmes*. Patient Liaison Group and General Practitioners Committee. www.bma.org.uk/ap.nsf/content/selfmanagementpolicy (accessed 3 June 2008).

BMA (2007b) *Health select committee – public and patient involvement in the NHS. Memorandum of evidence from the BMA's Patient Liaison Group*, 12 January. www.bma.org.uk/ap.nsf/content/ppnhs (accessed 29 May 2008).

Boseley, S. (2002) Drive to narrow health gap between rich and poor, *Guardian*, 15 April.

Bottomley, V. (1994) Government's role in promoting good health, *Sunday Times*, 21 August.

Bradley, E. and Nolan, P. (2007) Impact of nurse prescribing: a qualitative study, *Journal of Advanced Nursing*, 59(2): 120–8.

Brandis, S. (2000) The Australian Healthcare Agreement 1998–2003: implications and strategic direction for occupational therapists, *Australian Occupational Therapy Journal*, 47: 62–8.

Brindle, D. (1991) District cuts NHS-funded abortions, *Guardian*, 15 November.

Brindle, D. (1992) Whose lifeline is it anyway? *Guardian*, 29 April.

Brindle, D. (1995) Dorrell discounts NHS crisis report, *Guardian*, 20 September.

Brindle, D. (1997) Nursing: voices raised in unison, *Guardian*, 14 May.

Brown, R. (2002) The NHS: last act of a Greek tragedy? *British Medical Journal*, http://findarticles.com/p/articles/mi_m0999/is_7260_321/ai_66676946 (accessed 2 September 2008).

Browne, A. and Young, M. (2002) NHS reform: towards consensus. Adam Smith Institute. www.adamsmith.org/pdf/browne-paper-1.pdf (accessed 15 January 2005).

Budge, I., Crewe, I., McKay, D. and Newton, K. (1998) *The New British Politics*. Essex: Wesley Longman.

Burman, E., Chantier, K. and Batsieer, J. (2002) Service responses to South Asian women who attempt suicide or self-harm: challenges for service commissioning and delivery, *Critical Social Policy*, 22: 641–68.

Bury, M. (1996) Defining and researching disability, in C. Barnes and G. Mercer (eds) *Exploring the Divide*. Leeds: The Disability Press.

Busfield, J. (2000) *Health and Health Care in Modern Britain*. Oxford: Oxford University Press.

Bush, G. (2004) *State of the Union Address*. www.whitehouse.gov/news/releases/2004/01/20040120-7.html (accessed 7 June 2008).

Caine, N., Sharples, L.D., Hollingworth, W. et al. (2002) A randomised controlled crossover trail of nurse practioner versus doctor led outpatient care in a bronchiectasis clinic, *Health Technology Assessment*, 6(27): 1–71.

Californian Department of Health Services (2001) Eliminating smoking in bars, taverns and gaming clubs: the Californian smoke-free workplace act. www.Cdph.Ca.Gov/Programs/Tobacco/Pages/Default.Aspx. (accessed 3 June 2008).

Californian Department of Industrial Relations (1995) *Labor Code Section 6404.5 Prohibiting Smoking In Places Of Employment*. www.Dir.State.Ca.Us (accessed 3 June 2008).

Cameron, A. (1999) The role of interest groups, in A. Masterson and S. Maslin-Prothero (eds) *Nursing and Politics*. Edinburgh: Churchill Livingstone, 115–42.

Campbell, C. and Rockman, B. (eds) (1996) *The Clinton Presidency*. New Jersey: Chatham House.

Canadian Population Health Initiative (2004) *Improving the Health of Canadians*. Ontario: Canadian Institute for Health Information. www.cihi.ca (accessed 3 June 2008).

Cannavina, C.D., Cannavina, G., Walsh, T.F. (2000) Effects of evidence-based treatment and consent on professional autonomy, *British Dental Journal*, 188(6): 302–6.

CBC News (2007) Ontario nurses condemn CMA's health-care plan, 31 July. www.cbc.ca/health/story/2007/07/31/nurses-privatehealth.html (accessed 3 June 2008).

Channel 4 (1998) *Pennies from Bevan*, 14 June.

CHO (2007) *Canadian Healthcare*. www.canadian-healthcare.org/index.html (accessed 3 December 2007).

Churchill, L. (1999) The United States health care system under managed care, *Health Care Analysis*, 7: 393–411.

Clarke, J. and Fox Piven, F. (2001) United States: An American Welfare State? in P. Alcock and G. Craig (eds) *International Social Policy*. Basingstoke: Palgrave, 26–44.

Colombo, F. and Tapay, N. (2003) *Private Health Insurance in Australia: A Case Study*. Paris: Organisation for Economic Co-operation and Development. www.oecd.org/document/48/0,3343,en_2649_34851_2088432_1_1_1_1,00.html (accessed 3 June 2008).

Conservative Party (1945) *Mr. Churchill's Declaration of Policy to the Electors*, Party Election Manifestos. www.psr.keele.ac.uk/area/uk/man/con45.htm (accessed 12 April 2008).

Conservative Party (1955) *United for Peace and Progress: The Conservative and Unionist Party's Policy*. Party Election Manifestos. www.psr.keele.ac.uk/area/uk/man/con55.htm (accessed 12 April 2008).

Conservative Party (1964) *Prosperity with a purpose*. Party Election Manifestos. www.psr.keele.ac.uk/area/uk/man/con64.htm (accessed 12 April 2008).

Conservative Party (1970a) *A Better Tomorrow*. February, Party Election Manifestos. www.psr.keele.ac.uk/area/uk/man/con70.htm (accessed 12 April 2008).

Conservative Party (1970b) *Putting Britain First*. Party Election Manifestos. www.psr.keele.ac.uk/area/uk/man/con74oct.htm (accessed 12 April 2008).

Conservative Party (1979) *Conservative Manifesto*. Party Election Manifestos. www.psr.keele.ac.uk/area/uk/man/con79.htm#health. (accessed 12 April 2008).

Conservative Party (1983) *Foreword – The Challenge of Our Times*. Party Election Manifestos. www.psr.keele.ac.uk/area/uk/man/con83.htm (accessed 12 April 2008).

Conservative Party (1987) *The Next Moves Forward*. Party Election Manifestos. www.psr.keele.ac.uk/area/uk/man/con87.htm (accessed 12 April 2008).

Conservative Party (1997) *You Can Only Be Sure With The Conservatives*. Party Election Manifestos. www.psr.keele.ac.uk/area/uk/man/con97.htm#health (accessed 12 April 2008).

Conservative Party (2007) *Stop Brown's NHS Cuts*. www.conservatives.com/tile.do?def=campaigns.display.page&obj_id=132788 (accessed 12 April 2008).

Cook, M. (2004) Should the voluntary sector be integral to public services? *Healthmatters*, 56(8): 10.

Crichton, A., Robertson, A., Gordon, C., Farrant, W. (1997) *Health Care: A Community Concern?* Calgary: University of Calgary.

Crosland, A. (1957) *The Future of Socialism*. New York: Macmillan.

Damms, R. (2002) *The Eisenhower Presidency*. London: Pearson Education.

Davey, B., Gray, A. and Seale, C. (1995) *Health and Disease: A Reader*. Buckingham: Open University Press.

Davis, S. (1999) A community development approach to health promotion, in M. Purdy and D. Banks (eds) *Health and Exclusion*. London: Routledge, 136–55.

Daykin, N. (2000) Sociology, in J. Naidoo and J. Wills (eds) *Health Studies: An Intro-duction*. Houndmills: Palgrave, 101–32.

Dean, M. (1996) Health: A ration of compassion, *Guardian*, 23 October.

Democratic Leadership Council (1991) *The New American Choice Resolutions*. Ohio: DLC Convention. www.dlc.org/ndol_ci.cfm?kaid=86&subid=194&contentid=1251 (accessed 12 April 2008).

Democrats (2001) The McCain-Edwards-Kennedy Patient Bill of Rights 1999 www.democrats.senate.gov/pbr/summary.html (accessed 3 June 2008).

Department of Health and Ageing (2008a) *Developing a Men's Health Policy for Australia: Setting the Scene*. www.health.gov.au/internet/main/publishing. nsf/Content/phd-mens-policy (accessed 2 April 2009).

Department of Health and Ageing (2008b) *Developing a Women's Health Policy for Australia: Setting the Scene*. Commonwealth of Australia. www.health.gov.au/internet/main/publishing.nsf/Content/F5D935422030AF1FCA25 75200072A29F/$File/women-brochure-dec08.pdf (accessed 2 April 2009).

Department of Health: New York State (2003) *Clean Indoor Air Act*. www.health. state.ny.us/nysdoh/clean_indoor_air_act/ciaalaw.htm. (accessed 2 June 2008).

Department of Human Services (2007) *The Oregon Health Plan*. www.oregon.gov/ DHS/healthplan/app_benefits/ohp4u.shtml (accessed 9 June 2008).

DH (Department of Health) (1991) *The Patient's Charter*. London: HMSO.

DH (1997) *The New NHS – Modern, Dependable*. London: Crown Copyright. www.archive.official-ocuments.co.uk/document/doh/newnhs/forward.htm (accessed 20 March 2008).

DH (1998) *The Acheson Report: Independent Inquiry into Inequalities in Health: Re-port*. London: Crown Copyright. www.dh.gov.uk/en/Publicationsandstatistics/ Publications/PublicationsPolicyAndGuidance/DH_4097582 (accessed 16 October 2009).

DH (1998b) *Modernising Mental Health Services: Safe, Sound and Supportive*. London: Crown Copyright.

DH (1999) *Tougher Regulation For Private Healthcare*. www.dh.gov.uk/en/ Publicationsandstatistics/Pressreleases/DH_4025843 (accessed 20 March 2008).

DH (2000) *The NHS Plan: A Plan for Investment, A Plan for Reform*. London: Crown Copyright.

DH (2001a) *The Report of the Chief Medical Officer's Project to Strengthen the Public Health Function*. London: HMSO.

DH (2001b) *Making it Happen: A Guide to Delivering Mental Health Promotion*. London: Crown Copyright.

DH (2001c) *The Mental Health Policy Implementation Guide*. London: Crown Copy-right.

DH (2001d) *The Journey to Recovery: The Government's Vision for Mental Health Care*. London: Crown Copyright.

DH (2001e) *The Expert Patient: A New Approach to Chronic Disease Management for the 21st Century.* London: Crown Copyright. www.dh.gov.uk/en/Publicationsandstatistics/Publications/PublicationsPolicyandGuidance/DH_400681 (accessed 16 October 2009).

DepartmentLeaders/ChiefMedicalOfficer/ProgressOnPolicy/ProgressBrowsable Document/DH_4102757 (accessed 20 March 2008).

DH (2002) *Health Check: Annual Report of The Chief Medical Officer.* London: DOH Publications.

DH (2003a) *The New NHS: Modern and Dependable,* in A. Chadwick and R. Hefferman (eds) *The New Labour Reader.* Cambridge: Polity, 149–54.

DH (2003b) *Choice, Responsiveness and Equity in the NHS.* London: Department of Health.

DH (2004a) *Choosing Health* (Command paper) www.dh.gov.uk/Publications AndStatistics/Publications/PublicationsPolicyAndGuidance/Publications PolicyAndGuidanceArticle/fs/en?CONTENT_ID=4094550&chk=aN5Cor (accessed 21 March 2008).

DH (2004b) *Getting Over the Wall.* www.dh.gov.uk/en/Publicationsandstatistics/Publications/PublicationsPolicyAndGuidance/DH_4090841 (accessed 21 March 2008).

DH (2005a) *Choosing Health: Making Healthier Choices Easier.* London: Crown Copyright.

DH (2005b) *Consultation on the Future Support for Patient and Public Involvement in Health: Report.* London.

DH (2005c) *Delivering Choosing Health: Making Healthier Choices Easier.* London: Crown Copyright.

DH (2005d) *Health Inequalities: Rising to the Challenge.* London: Health Inequalities Unit. www.dh.gov.uk/en/Publicationsandstatistics/Pressreleases/DH_4002603 (accessed 23 March 2008).

DH (2006a) *Our Health, Our Care, Our Say: A New Direction for Community Services.* London: Crown Copyright. www.dh.gov.uk/en/Policyandguidance/Organisationpolicy/Modernisation/Ourhealthourcareoursay/index.htm (accessed 23 March 2008).

DH (2006b) *Choosing Health: Supporting the Physical Health Needs of People with Severe Mental Illness.* London: Crown Copyright. http://www.dh.gov.uk/en/Publicationsandstatistics/Publications/PublicationsPolicyAndGuidance/DH_4138212 (accessed 5 January 2008).

DH (2007a) *Equity, Equality and Health Policy: Rationing.* Healthknowledge – The online resource for Public Health Practioners. www.healthknowledge.org.uk/index.html (accessed 15 April 2008).

DH (2007b) *Everything You Need to Prepare for the New Smoke Free Law on July 1st 2007.* London: DH Publications.

DH (2008a) *Health Inequalities.* London: Crown Copyright. www.dh.gov.uk/en/Policyandguidance/Healthandsocialcaretopics/Healthinequalities/index.htm (accessed 5 July 2008).

DH (2008b) *Patient and Public Involvement.* www.dh.gov.uk/en/Managingyour organisation/PatientAndPublicinvolvement/index.htm (accessed 6 May 2008).

DH (2008c) *The Gender and Access to Health Service Study: Final Report.* London: Crown Copyright.

DH (2008d) *High Quality Care for All. NHS Next Stage Review, Final report.* London: Crown Copyright.

DH (2009) What is PALS www.pals.nhs.uk/cmsContentView.aspx?ItemID=932 (accessed 24 March 2009).

DHSSPS (2002) *Investing for Health.* Belfast: Crown Copyright. www.dhsspni.gov.uk/show_publications?txtid=10415 (accessed 10 October 2009).

Dillon, J. (2001) Focus: National health – the nurses: higher expectations can't all be delivered, *Independent on Sunday,* 2 December.

Dixon, A. and Le Grand, J. (2006) Is greater patient choice consistent with equity? The case of the English NHS, *Journal of Health Service Research Policy,* 11(3): 162–6.

Downs, M. and Bowers, B. (2008) Caring for people with dementia, *British Medical Journal,* Editorials, 336: 225–6.

Drake, R. (1999) *Understanding Disability Politics.* Houndmills: Macmillan.

Dranove, D. (2000) *The Economic Evolution of American Health Care: From Marcus Welby to Managed Care.* Princeton: Princeton University Press.

Emanuel, L., Cruess, R., Cruess, S. and Hauser, J. (2002) Old values, new challenges: what is a professional to do? *International Journal for Quality in Health Care,* 14(5): 349–51.

Embassy of Spain (1995) *The National Health Institute (Insalud),* 'Si Spain'. www.sispain.org/english/health/helintro.html (accessed 6 January 2008).

European Commission (2006) *Mental Health Promotion and Mental Disorder Prevention Across European Member States.* www.ec.europa.eu/health/ph_projects/2004/action1/docs/action1_2004_a02_30_en.pdf (accessed 18 February 2008).

European Commission (2007) *Closing the Gap: Strategies for Action to Tackle Health Inequalities.* www.health-inequalities.org/?uid=408ced42eb9051c40aac6291b0e 836f9&id=Seite2113 (accessed 17 January 2008).

Ewles, L. and Simnett, I. (1985) *Promoting Health.* Chichester: Wiley.

Farrell, C. (1999) The Patients Charter: a tool for quality improvement? *International Journal of Health Care Quality Assurance,* 12(4): 129–34.

Farrell, C. (2004) *Patient and Public Involvement in Health: The Evidence for Policy Implementation.* London: DH.

Fatchett, A. (1994) *Politics, Policy and Nursing.* London: Balliere Tindall.

Fatchett, A. (1998) *Nursing in the New NHS.* London: Bailliere Tindall.

Feek, C., McKean, M., Henneveld, L., Barrow, E.W., Edgar, W. and Paterson, R. (1999) Experience with Rationing health care in New Zealand, *British Medical Journal,* 318(7194): 1346–48.

Fitzpatrick, M. (2001) *The Tyranny of Health.* London: Routledge.

Fitzpatrick, M. and Milligan, D. (1987) *The Truth About the AIDS Panic*. London: Janus.

Fletcher, D. (1994) Give elderly equal treatment, *The Telegraph*, 11 May.

Fletcher, D. (1996) Health rationing on the increase, *The Telegraph*, 6 June.

Flood, C. (2000) *International Health Care Reform*. London: Routledge.

Forster, R. and Gabe, J. (2008) Voice or choice? Patient and public involvement in the National Health Service in England under New Labour, *International Journal of Health Services*, 38(2): 333–56.

Friedman, M. (1962) *Capitalism and Freedom*. Chicago: The University of Chicago Press.

Fuller, J. (1995) Challenging old notions of professionalism: how can nurses work with paraprofessional ethnic health workers? *Journal of Advanced Nursing*, 22: 465–72.

Furler, J., Harris, E., Harris, M. et al. (2007) Health Inequalities, physician citizens and professional medical associations: an Australian case study, *BMC Medicine*, 5: 23.

Gampel, E. (2006) Does professional autonomy protect medical futility judgements? *Bioethics*, 20(2): 92–104.

Gerrish, K., McManus, M. and Ashworth, P. (2003) Creating what sort of professional? *Nursing Inquiry*, 10: 103–12.

Giddens, A. (2000) *The Third Way and its Critics*. Cambridge: Polity.

Gillespie, G. and Gerhardt, C. (1995) Social dimensions of sickness and disability, in G. Moon and R. Gillespie (eds) *Society and Health*. London: Routledge, 75–96.

Gillespie, R. and Prior, R. (1995) Health inequalities, in G. Moon and R. Gillespie (eds) *Society and Health*. London: Routledge, 195–212.

Gilmour, I. (1992) *Dancing with Dogma*. London: Pocket Books. (1993 reprint)

Ginsburg, N. (1992) *Divisions of Welfare*. London: Sage.

Glennerster, H. (2000) *British Social Policy since 1945*. Oxford: Blackwell.

Goldby, F.S. (2002) The NHS: last act of a Greek tragedy? *British Medical Journal*, 2 Sept. www. findarticles.com/p/articles/mi_m0999/is_7260_321/ai_66676946 (accessed 9 June 2008).

Goodyear-Smith, F. and Buetow, S. (2001) Power issues in the doctor–patient relationship, *Health Care Analysis*, 9: 449–62.

Gorz, A. (1980) *Ecology as Politics*. London: Pluto Press.

Gott, M. and O'Brien, M. (1990) The role of the nurse in health promotion, *Health Promotion International*, 5(2): 137–43.

Gould, A. (1993) *Capitalist Welfare Systems*. London: Longman.

Government of Canada (2002) *Patient Bill of Rights – A Comparative Overview. Law and Government Division*. www.dsp-psd.pwgsc.gc.ca/Collection-R/LoPBdP/ BP/prb0131-e.htm (accessed 4 April 2008).

Graham, H. (1997) Health: poverty is a deadly disease, *Guardian*, 25 June.

Graham, H. and Kelly, M. (2004) *Health Inequalities: Concepts, Frameworks and Policy*.

Health Development Agency. www.hda-online.org.uk/Documents/health_inequalities_concepts.pdf (accessed 15 January 2005).

Green, D. (1995) Why it's time to dismantle the NHS, *Evening Standard*, 20 September.

Green, J. (2006) New professionalism in the 21st Century, *The Lancet.* 367(9511): 646–7.

Green Party (2000) *Manifesto for a Sustainable Society: Health.* www.greenparty. org.uk/policy/mfss/health.html (accessed 6 June 2001).

Gubb, J. (2008) Should patients be able to pay top up fees to receive the treatment that they want? Yes, *BMJ*, 336: 1104.

Guglielmo, W.J. (2004) Why Oregon's rationing plan is gasping for air. *Medical Economics.* medicaleconomics.modernmedicine.com/memag/article/article Detail.jsp?id=127172&sk=&date=&%0A%09%09%09&pageID=2 (accessed 5 May 2008).

Ham, C. (1992) *Health Policy in Britain.* Houndmills: Macmillan.

Hansard (2000) *Cosmetic Surgery.* May 10, cols 201–21. London: HMSO. www. publications.parliament.uk/pa/cm199900/cmhansrd/vo000510/halltext/ 00510h01.htm (accessed 9 May 2008).

Hansard (2001) *Private Finance Initiative.* Vol. 372, part no. 22, cols 1–135. London: HMSO. www.publications.parliament.uk/pa/cm200102/cmhansrd/ vo010717/hallindx/10717-x.htm (accessed 9 May 2008).

Hansard (2002) *Finance Bill.* Vol. 388, part no. 170, cols 247–372. www.parliament. the-stationery-office.co.uk/pa/cm200102/cmhansrd/vo020703/debindx/ 20703-x.htm (accessed 9 May 2008).

Harris, E. (1999) Is competition good for medicine? *Health Care Analysis*, 7: 91–8.

Hastings, C. and Fraser, L. (2001) 20,000 NHS nurses opt for private health cover, *The Telegraph.* www.telegraph.co.uk (accessed 10 June 2008).

Hausman, D., Asada, Y. and Hedemann, T. (2002) Health inequalities and why they matter, *Health Care Analysis*, 10: 177–91.

Hayek, F. (1960) *The Constitution of Liberty.* London: Routledge and Kegan Paul.

Health and Medical Development Advisory Committee (2005a) *Landscape on Health Care Services in Hong Kong.* www.fhb.gov.hk/hmdac/english/dis_papers/ dis_papers_lhcshk.html (accessed 20 April 2008).

Health and Medical Development Advisory Committee (2005b) *Building a Healthy Tomorrow – Discussion Paper on Future Service Delivery: Model for our Health Care System.* www.fhb.gov.hk/hmdac/english/dis_papers/dis_papers.html (accessed 2 April 2008).

Health Canada (1999) *Women's Health Strategy.* www.hc-sc.gc.ca/ahc-asc/pubs/ strateg-women-femmes/strateg-eng.php (accessed 9 March 2009).

Health Canada (2003) *Exploring Concepts of Gender and Health.* Ottawa: Women's Health Bureau. www.hc-sc.gc.ca/hl-vs/pubs/women-femmes/explor-eng.php (accessed 9 March 2009).

Health Canada (2005) *Canada's Health Care System*. Her Majesty the Queen in Right of Canada. www.hc-sc.gc.ca/hcs-sss/pubs/system-regime/2005-hcs-sss/index_e.html (accessed 6 January 2008).

Health Canada (2006) *Canada Health Act: Annual Report, 2005–2006*. Ontario: Minister of Health Canada. www.healthcanada.ag.ca/medicare (accessed 6 January 2008).

Health Canada (2007) *People with Disabilities*. http://www.hc-sc.gc.ca/jfy-spv/disinca_e.html (accessed 16 October 2009).

Health Canada (2008) *Canada's Health Care System (Medicare)*. www.hc-sc.gc.ca/hcs-sss/medi-assur/index_e.html (accessed 6 January 2008).

Health Development Agency (2004) *The Effectiveness of Public Health Campaigns*. London.

Health Disparities Task Group of the Federal/Provincial/Territorial Advisory Committee on Population Health and Health Security (2004) *Reducing Health Disparities – Roles of the Health Sector: Discussion Paper*. Her Majesty the Queen in Right of Canada, represented by the Minister of Health. www.phac-aspc.gc.ca/ph-sp/disparities/ddp_e.html (accessed 8 April 2008).

Health and Welfare Canada (1986) *Achieving Health for All: A Framework for Health Promotion*. www.hc-sc.gc.ca/hcs-sss/pubs/system-regime/1986-frame-plan-promotion/index_e.html (accessed 16 October 2009).

Hill, M. (1997) *Understanding Social Policy*. Oxford: Blackwell.

HM Treasury (2007) *Public Private Partnerships: The Private Finance Initiative (PFI)*. www.hm-treasury.gov.uk/documents/public_private_partnerships/ppp_index.cfm (accessed 3 April 2008).

HM Treasury (2006) *PFI: Strengthening Long-Term Partnerships*. Norwich: Crown Copyright. www.hm-treasury.gov.uk/budget/budget_06/other_documents/bud_bud06_odpfi.cfm (accessed 3 April 2008).

Hoedemaekers, R. and Dekkers, W. (2003) Justice and solidarity in priority setting in health care, *Health Care Analysis*, 11: 325–49.

Holm, S., Liss, P. and Norheim, O. (1999) Access to health care in Scandinavia Countries: ethical aspects, *Health Care Analysis*, 7: 321–30.

House of Commons (2001) *Health: Second Report*. HMSO: London.

Houtepen, R. and Muelen, R. (2000) The expectation(s) of solidarity: matters of justice, responsibility and identity in the reconstruction of the health care system, *Health Care Analysis*, 8: 355–76.

Human Rights and Equal Opportunities Commission (2008) *Gender Equality: What Matters to Australian Men and Women*. Sydney. www.humanrights.gov.au (accessed 28 March 2009).

Hutton, J. (2004) *The Government and the Private Sector*. Department of Health www.dh.gov.uk/NewsHome/Speeches/SpeechesList/SpeechesArticle/fs/en?CONTENT_ID=4083816&chk=s1KCfL (accessed 18 January 2005).

Institute of Medicine (2002) *Unequal Treatment: What Healthcare Providers Need to Know About Racial and Ethnic Disparities in Health Care*. National Academy of Sciences. www.nap.edu (accessed 17 March 2008).

Intute (2008) *Hot topic: Prescribing by Nurses, Midwives and Allied Health Professionals.* www.intute.ac.uk/healthandlifesciences/hottopic_39.html (accessed 7 July 2008).

Irish Patients Association (2002) *Healthcare Rights and Responsibilities: A Review of the European Charter of Patient Rights.* Dublin. www.dcu.ie/nursing/healthcare_rights.shtml (accessed 6 January 2008).

Irvine, D. (2001) Doctors in the U.K: their new professionalism and its regulatory framework, *Lancet,* 358: 1807–10.

Jones, J. (1993) Health rationing comes into the open after patient dies, *The Independent,* 7 March.

Jones, L. (1994) *The Social Context of Health and Health Work.* Houndmills: Macmillan.

Kane, K. (2008) Case finding in the community: the results 2, *British Journal of Community Nursing,* 13(6): 265–9.

Kavanagh, D. (1994) A Major agenda, in D. Kavanagh and A. Seldon (eds) *The Major Effect.* London: Macmillan.

Kennedy, C. (2001) *The Future of Politics.* London: Harper Collins.

Kent, A. (1998) Few patients are aware of content of patients charter. *British Medical Journal,* 317: 1543.

Kirk, S. (2004) Agenda for change: implications for the voluntary sector, *Nursing Management,* 11(1): 16–8.

Klein, R. (1993) Dimensions of rationing: who should do what? *British Medical Journal,* 307: 309–11.

Klein, R. (2001) *The New Politics of the National Health Service.* Harlow: Prentice Hall.

Labour Party (1950) *Let Us Win Through Together: A Declaration of Labour Policy for the Consideration of the Nation.* Party Election Manifestos. www.psr.keele.ac.uk/area/uk/man/lab50.htm (accessed 12 April 2008).

Labour Party (1964) *The New Britain.* Party Election Manifestos. www.psr.keele.ac.uk/area/uk/man/lab64.htm (accessed 12 April 2008).

Labour Party (1966) *Time for Decision.* Party Election Manifestos. www.psr.keele.ac.uk/area/uk/man/lab66.htm (accessed 12 April 2008).

Labour Party (1979) *The Labour Way is the Better Way.* Party Election Manifestos. www.psr.keele.ac.uk/area/uk/man/lab79.htm (accessed 12 April 2008).

Labour Party (1983) *The New Hope for Britain.* Party Election Manifestos. www.psr.keele.ac.uk/area/uk/man/lab83.htm (accessed 12 April 2008).

Labour Party (1987) *Britain Will Win with Labour.* Party Election Manifestos. www.psr.keele.ac.uk/area/uk/man/lab87.htm (accessed 12 April 2008).

Labour Party (1992) *It's Time to Get Britain Working Again.* Party Election Manifestos. www.psr.keele.ac.uk/area/uk/man/lab92.htm#nhs (accessed 12 April 2008).

Le Grand, J. (2001) *The Provision of Health Care: Is the Public Sector Ethically Superior to the Private Sector?* LSE Health and Social Care Discussion Paper Number 1. London. www.lse.ac.uk/collections/LSEHealthAndSocialCare/pdf/DiscussionPaperSeries/DP1_2002.pdf (accessed 15 January 2005).

Liberal/SDP Alliance (1983) *Working Together for Britain*. Party Election Manifestos. www.psr.keele.ac.uk/area/uk/man/all83.htm (accessed 12 April 2008).

Liberal/SDP Alliance (1987) *Britain United: The Time Has Come*. www.psr.keele.ac.uk/area/uk/man/lib87.htm (accessed 12 April 2008).

Light, D.W. (1997) *The Real Ethics of Rationing, British Medical Journal*, 315: 112–15.

Lincoln, P. and Nutbeam, D. (2006) What is health promotion? in M. Davies and W. Macdowall (eds) *Health Promotion Theory*. Maidenhead: Open University Press, 7–15.

Linder, S. and Rosenau, P. (2002) Health care policy, in G. Peele, C. Bailey, B. Cain and B.G. Peters (eds) *Developments in American Politics 4*. Houndmills: Palgrave, 222–33.

Lloyd, L. (2001) Social policy, in J. Naidoo and J. Wills (eds) *Health Studies: An Introduction*. Houndmills: Palgrave, 163–92.

Loewy, E.H. (1999) Health care systems and ethics: what can we learn? *Health Care Analysis*, 7: 309–20.

Marks, D. (1999) *Disability*. London: Routledge.

Maslin-Prothero, S. and Masterson, A. (1999) Power, politics and nursing, in A. Masterson and S. Maslin-Prothero (eds) *Nursing and Politics*. Edinburgh: Churchill Livingstone, 209–31.

McGarry, J. (2003) The essence of community within community nursing and district nursing perspective, *Health and Social Care in the Community*, 11: 423–30.

McQueen, D. (2002) Discomfort of patient power, *British Medical Journal*, 18 May. www.bmj.com/cgi/content/extract/324/7347/1214 (accessed 7 June 2008).

McRae, H. (1994) Health care rationing comes into the open, *The Independent*, 26 May.

Medical Research Council (2007) *Inequalities in Health in Scotland: What are They and What Can we Do About Them?* Glasgow: MRC Social and Public Health Sciences Unit. www.sphsu.mrc.ac.uk (accessed 19 March 2008).

Ministry of Health (2001) *The New Zealand Disability Strategy: Making a World of Difference*. Wellington: Ministry of Health. www.odi.govt.nz/publications/nzds/index.html (accessed 9 April 2008).

Ministry of Health (2005) *Implementing Nurse Practitioner Prescribing*. Consultation document. Wellington: MOH. http://www.nurse.org.nz/nurse_practitioner/consultation.pdf (accessed 4 November 2005).

Ministry of Health (2006) *Implementing the New Zealand Health Strategy 2006: The Minister of Health's Sixth Report on the New Zealand Health Strategy*. Wellington: Ministry of Health. www.moh.govt.nz/moh.nsf/pagesmh/5651/$File/implementing-nz-health-strategy-2006.pdf (accessed 2 June 2008).

Ministry of Health (2008) *Men's Health*. www.moh.govt.nz/menshealth (accessed 28 March 2009).

Mirchandani, R. (2008) *Oregon's Healthcare Lottery*. BBC News. Oregon. 30 March. www.news.bbc.co.uk/2/hi/health/7321500.stm (accessed 4 July 2008).

Mollar, P. and Begg, E. (2005) Independent nurse prescribing in New Zealand, *Journal of New Zealand Medical Association*, 18: 1225.

Moroney, R.M. and Krysik, J. (1998) *Social Policy and Social Work*. New York: Aldine de Gruyter.

Morris, J. (1993) Gender and disability, in J. Swain, V. Finkelstein, S. French and M. Oliver (1993) *Disabling Barriers and Enabling Environments*. London: Sage, 85–93.

Morris, Z. (2001) Treatment must be rationed for NHS to survive, *Evening Standard*, 6 February.

Murray, I. (1998) Nurses told to challenge poor levels of care, *The Times*, 23 April.

Naidoo, J. and Wills, J. (2000) *Health Promotion*. Edinburgh: Bailliere Tindall.

National Health Committee (2004) *Prioritising Health Services*. www.nhc.govt.nz (accessed 11 June 2008).

National Prescribing Centre (2004) *MeReC Briefing: Supplementary Prescribing*. Issue no. 23. Liverpool. www.npc.co.uk (accessed 11 June 2008).

New York City Department of Health and Mental Hygiene (2004) *Health Disparities in New York City*. New York: Fund for Public Health in New York inc. www.nyc.gov/html/doh//downloads/pdf/epi/disparities-2004.pdf (accessed 5 April 2008).

New York City Health (2007) *Smoke Free Workplace Legislation Will Save Lives And Won't Hurt Businesses*. www.Nyc.Gov/Html/Doh/Html/Smoke/Tc1.Shtml (accessed 9 May 2008).

New York State Department of Health (2004) *Women's Health Programs in New York State*. www.health.state.ny.us/community/adults/women/womens_health_directory/index.htm (accessed 25 March 2009).

NHS Direct Wales (2008) Useful Patient Information. www.nhsdirect.wales.nhs.uk/small/en/home/healthinformation/usefulpatientinformation (accessed 7 June 2008).

NHSCCA (1990) *National Health Service and Community Care Act*. www.opsi.gov.uk/acts/acts1990/ukpga_19900019_en_1#Legislation-Preamble (accessed 18 January 2008).

NHS Scotland (2000) *Our National Health: A Plan for Action, A Plan for Change*. Crown Copyright. www.scotland.gov.uk/Resource/Doc/158732/0043081.pdf. (accessed 2 April 2008).

NHS Scotland (2003a) *Supplementary Prescribing by Nurses Within NHS Scotland: A Guide for Implementation*. Scottish Executive Health Department. Edinburgh: Crown Copyright.

NHS Scotland (2003b) *Patient Rights and Responsibilities: A Draft for Consultation*. Edinburgh: Crown Copyright.

NHS Scotland (2008) *Latest Research + Expert Opinion + Patient Experience= Better Healthcare*. www.nhshealthquality.org/nhsqis/37.140.141.html (accessed 2 April 2008).

NIMHE (National Institute for Mental Health in England) (2003) *Inside Out: Improving Mental Health Services for Black and Ethnic Communities in England.* www.nimhe.org.uk (accessed 4 December 2007).

Nixon, R. (1971) *Special Message to the Congress Proposing a National Health Strategy*, 18 February. www.nixonfoundation.org/Research_Center/ (accessed 19 May 2008).

Nordenfelt, L. (2001) On the goals of medicine, health enhancement and social welfare, *Health Care Analysis*, 9: 15–23.

North, N. (1995) Managing the NHS, in G. Moon and G. Gillespie (eds) *Health and Society*. London: Routledge, 181–94.

North, N. (2001) Health policy, in S. Savage and R. Atkinson (eds) *Public Policy Under Blair*. Houndmills: Palgrave, 123–38.

NP Canada (2007) *Welcome to NPCanada.ca*, 25 March. www.npcanada.ca/portal/ (accessed 5 February 2008).

Nursing in Practice (2006) Public health: The role of the district nurse, 31. www.nursinginpractice.com/default.asp? (accessed 4 June 2008).

Nursing in Practice (2008) Nurses could run NHS businesses, 27 June. www.nursinginpractice.com/default.asp?title=NursescouldrunNHS%22businesses%22&page=article.display&article.id=12006 (accessed 4 June 2008).

Obama, B. and Biden, J. (2009) Plan for a healthy America: Barack Obama and Joe Biden's Plan. http://www.barackobama.com/issues/healthcare (accessed 20 April 2009).

O'Connor-Fleming, M.L. and Parker, E. (2001) *Health Promotion Principles and Practice in the Australian Context*. New South Wales: Allen and Unwin.

Olthuis, G. and Van Heteren, G. (2003) Multicultural health care in practice: an empirical exploration of multicultural care in the Netherlands, *Health Care Analysis*, 11: 199–206.

Palfrey, C. (2000) *Key Concepts in Health Care Policy and Planning*. Houndmills: Macmillan.

Palmer, A. (1996) Focus- health service rationing, *The Telegraph*, 14 April.

Parker, G. and Suzman, M. (1995) Dorrell seeks £400 million to weed out useless cures, *Financial Times*, 28 September.

Peckham, S. and Meerabeau, L. (2007) *Social Policy for Nurses and the Helping Professions*. Maidenhead: Open University Press.

Perkins, E. (1999) An introduction to political perspectives, in A. Masterson and S. Maslin-Prothero (eds) *Nursing and Politics*. Edinburgh: Churchill Livingstone, 37–71.

Pike, A. (1991) Criticism mounts over NHS reforms, *The Financial Times*, 13 May.

Pike, A. (1992) Doctors open the debate on care rationing, *The Financial Times*, 7 July.

Pilkington, E. (1995) Abortion cut-back will hit teenagers, *Guardian*, 28 October.

Porritt, J. (1984) *Seeing Green*. London: Blackwell.

PPP Forum (2007) Labour Party Policy on PPI. www.ppp.squareeye.com/government/article.asp?p=263.~ (accessed 23 June 2007).

Prechel, H. and Gupman, A. (1995) Changing economic conditions and their effects on professional autonomy: an analysis of family practitioners and oncologists, *Sociological Forum*, 10(2): 245–71.

Presidents New Freedom Commission on Mental Health (2003) *Achieving the Promise: Transforming Mental Health Care in America*. www.mentalhealth commission.gov./ (accessed 12 December 2007).

Prime Ministers Strategy Unit (2005) *Improving the Life Chances of Disabled People*. London: Crown Copyright.

Propper, C., Wilson, D. and Burgess, S. (2006) Extending choice in English health-care: the implications of the economic evidence, *The Journal of Social Policy*, 35(4): 537–57.

Ranade, W. (1997) *A Future for the NHS?* London: Longman.

Reid, J. (2004a) *Choosing Health – Closing the Gap on Inequalities*. Department of Health. www.dh.gov.uk/NewsHome/Speeches/SpeechesList/SpeechesArticle/fs/en?CONTENT_ID=4081307&chk=96zwcE (accessed 26 November 2007).

Reid, J. (2004b) Speech to the faculty of Public Health, 10 June, Department of Health.

Reid, J. and Phillips, T. (2004) Society: Comment special: Different strokes, *Guardian*, 14 July.

Republican Party (2007) *State of the Union Address*. Republican National Committee, 23 January. www.gop.com/news/NewsRead.aspx?Guid=59f1d879-b99a-4c13-84c7-83f5ed070f1d (accessed 15 January 2008).

Roberts, R., Towell, T. and Golding, J. (2001) *Foundations of Health Psychology*. Basingstoke: Palgrave.

Rogers, W. (2002) Whose autonomy? Which choice? A study of GP attitudes towards patient autonomy in the management of low back pain, *Family Practice*, 19(2): 140–5.

Ross, F. and MacKenzie, A. (1996) *Nursing in Primary Health Care*. London: Routledge.

Rothman, D. (2001) The origins and consequences of patient autonomy: a 25 year retrospective, *Health Care Analysis*, 9: 255–64.

Royal College of Physicians (2005) *Doctors in Society: Medical Professionalism in a Changing World*. Report of a working party of the Royal College of Physicians of London. London: RCP.

Royal College of Radiologists (2005) *Tackling Health Inequalities*. London: Royal College of Radiologists. www.rcr.ac.uk/docs/radiology/pdf/WEBhealth inequalities.pdf (accessed 4 January 2008).

Sampson, V. (2000) Is private care bad for your health? *The Times*, 5 December.

Scottish Executive (2003) *National Programme for Improving Mental Health and Well-being: Action plan 2003–2006*. www.scotland.gov.uk/Publications/2003/09/18193/26508 (accessed 2 March 2008).

Scottish Executive (2005) *Smoke-Free Scotland: Guidance on Smoking Policies for the NHS, Local Authorities and Care Service Providers*. www.Scotland.Gov.Uk/Publications/2005/12/21153341 (accessed 4 January 2008).

Scottish Executive (2006a) *Delivering Care, Enabling Health: Harnessing the Nursing, Midwifery and Allied Health Professions' Contribution to Implementing Delivering for Health in Scotland.* www.scotland.gov.uk/Publications/2006/10/23103937/2 (accessed 2 March 2008).

Scottish Executive (2006b) *Delivering a Healthier Scotland: Meeting the Challenge.* Edinburgh: Crown Copyright. www.scotland.gov.uk/Publications/2006/11/29141927 (accessed 2 March 2008).

Scottish Office (1999) *Towards a Healthier Scotland. A White Paper on Health.* www.scotland.gov.uk/library/documents-w7/tahs-00.htm (accessed 2 March 2008).

Scottish Parliament (2006) *Equal Opportunities Committee Report: Removing Barriers and Creating Opportunities*, 2nd report. www.scottish.parliament.uk/business/committees/equal/reports-06/eor06-02-Vol01-00.htm (accessed 2 March 2008).

Sebelius, K. (2009) Remarks by president Obama, his secretary-designate Kathleen Sebelius, and white house office of health reform director Nancy-Ann Deparle, The White House, Office of the Press Secretary. www.whitehouse.gov/the_press_office/Remarks-by-President-Obama-HHS-Secretary-designate-Kathleen-Sebelius-and-White-Hou/ (accessed 11 June 2009).

Senior, M. and Viveash, B. (1998) *Health and Illness.* Houndmills: Palgrave.

Shaw, M., Dorling, D., Davey Smith, G. et al. (1999) Poverty, social exclusion and minorities, in M. Marmot and R. Wilkinson (eds) *Social Determinants of Health.* Oxford: Oxford University Press, 211–33.

Sheaf, R. (1996) *The Need for Health Care.* London: Routledge.

Silove, D. (2004) The global challenge of asylum, in D. Wilson and B. Drozdek (eds) *Broken Spirits: The Treatment of Traumatized Asylum Seekers, Refugees and Torture Victims.* London: Routledge, 13–32.

Smith, N. (2005a) Midwives not to blame for the state of healthcare, *British Journal of Midwifery*, Editorial, 13(8): 476–8.

Smith, N. (2005b) Midwives can help to reduce health inequalities, *British Journal of Midwifery*, Editorial, September 13(9): 540–2.

Sontag, S. (1978) Illness as metaphor, in B. Davey, A. Gray and C. Seale (eds) *Health and Disease: A Reader.* Buckingham: Open University Press, 33–7.

Sorell, T. (2001) Citizen-patient/citizen-doctor, *Health Care Analysis*, 9: 25–39.

Status of Women in Canada (1995) Setting the stage for the next century: the federal plan for gender equality. Ottawa. www.dsp-psd.pwgsc.gc.ca/Collection/SW21-15-1995E.pdf (accessed 28 March 2009).

Stewart, S. (1999) Cost-containment and privatisation: an international analysis, in D. Drache and T. Sullivan (eds) *Market Limits in Health Reform.* London: Routledge, 65–84.

Strategic Inter-Governmental Nutrition Alliance of the National Public Health Partnership 2000–2010 (2001) *Eat Well Australia: An Agenda for Action for Public*

Health Nutrition www.health.gov.au/internet/main/publishing.nsf/Content/ health-pubhlth-strateg-food-nphp.htm (accessed 10 April 2009).

Suzman, M. (1995) Think-tank report calls for extended private care, *Financial Times*, 20 September.

Suzman, M. (1997) Health service managers urge reform of PFI, *Financial Times*, 22 April.

Swedish National Institute of Public Health (2008) *Health for All? A Critical Analysis of Public Health Policies in Eight European Countries.* Stockholm. www.health-inequalities.eu/ (accessed 2 April 2009).

Tauber, A. (2001) Historical and philosophical reflections on patient autonomy, *Health Care Analysis*, 9: 299–319.

Taylor, C. (1979) What's wrong with negative liberty? In A. Ryan (ed.) *The Idea of Freedom.* Oxford: Oxford University Press, 175–93.

Taylor, G. (1999) *The State and Social Policy.* Sheffield: Sheffield Hallam University Press.

Taylor, G. (2007) *Ideology and Welfare.* London: Palgrave Macmillan.

Taylor, G. and Hawley, H. (2004) The construction of arguments over the rationing of health care, *The Social Policy Journal*, 3(3): 45–62.

Taylor, G. and Hawley, H. (2006) Health promotion and the freedom of the individual, *Health Care Analysis*, 14: 15–24.

Thatcher, M. (1984) *Speech to Conservative Party Conference: Conference Centre.* Brighton. www.margaretthatcher.org/speeches/displaydocument.asp?docid= 105763 (accessed 5 March 2008).

Theurl, E. (1999) Some aspects of the reform of the health care systems in Austria, Germany and Switzerland, *Health Care Analysis*, 7: 331–54.

Thompson, N. and Hammer, M. (2007) Weaving gold: transitioning nursing practice from a medical model to a nursing model, Oncology Nursing Forum, 34(2): 483.

Thomson, S. and Mossialos, E. (2004) *Funding Health Care from Private Sources: What are the Implications for Equity, Efficiency, Cost Containment and Choice in Western European Health Systems?* Copenhagen: World Health Organizational Regional Office for Europe.

Thomson, S. and Mossialos, E. (2006) *Regulating Private Health Insurance in the European Union: The Implications of Single Market Legislation and Competition Policy.* London: LSE Health. www.lse.ac.uk/collections/LSEHealth/pdf/ LSEHealthworkingpaperseries/LSEHWP4.pdf (accessed 2 June 2008).

Timmins, N. (1995) A suitable case for treatment: the future of the NHS, *The Independent*, 12 June.

Titmus, R. (1968) *Commitment to Welfare.* New York: Pantheon Books.

Todd, M. and Taylor, G. (2004) (eds) *Democracy and Participation.* London: Merlin Press.

Todd, M. and Ware, P. (2001) *The Voluntary Sector.* Sheffield: Sheffield Hallam University Press.

Tramior, J., Pomeroy, E. and Pope, B. A. (2004) *A Framework for Support*, 3rd edn. Toronto: Canadian Mental Health Association.

United States Department of Health (2001) *Healthy People in Healthy Communities*. Washington: ODPHP.

US Department of Health and Human Services (1999) www.hhs.gov/news/press/1999pres/9904 12.html (accessed 15 October 2009).

US Department of Health and Human Services (2000a) *Healthy People 2010: The Cornerstone for Prevention*. www.healthypeople.gov/Publications/Cornerstone. pdf (accessed 3 October 2007).

US Department of Health and Human Services (2000b) *Healthy People 2010: Understanding and Improving Health*. US Government Printing Office. www. healthypeople.gov/Document/tableofcontents.htm#under (accessed 3 October 2007).

US Department of Health and Human Services (2001) *National Strategy for Suicide Prevention*. www.mentalhealth.samhsa.gov/suicideprevention/strategy.asp (accessed 3 October 2007).

US Department of Health and Human Services (2003) *The Power of Prevention*. www. healthierus.gov/STEPS/summit/prevportfolio/power/index.html (accessed 3 October 2007).

US Department of Health and Human Services (2004) *Mental Health, United States*. www.mentalhealth.samhsa.gov/publications/allpubs/sma05-4018/ (accessed 3 October 2007).

US Department of Health and Human Services (2005a) *The Surgeon General's Call to Action to Improve the Health and Wellness of Persons with Disabilities*. www. surgeongeneral.gov/ (accessed 3 October 2007).

US Department of Health and Human Services (2005b) *Community Integration for Older Adults with Mental Illnesses: Overcoming Barriers and Seizing Opportunities*. www.mentalhealth.samhsa.gov/publications/allpubs/sma05-4018/ (accessed 3 October 2007).

US Department of Health and Human Services (2007a) *Healthy People10*. www. healthypeople.gov/Implementation/default.htm#partners (accessed 12 December 2007).

US Department of Health and Human Services (2007b) *Value-Driven Health Care Home*. www.hhs.gov/valuedriven/index.html (accessed 12 December 2007).

US Department of Health and Human Services (2009) The Presidents 2009 Budget. Office of Management and Budget. www.whitehouse.gov/omb/budget/fy2009/hhs.html (accessed 30 May 2009).

US Public Health Service (1999) *The First Surgeon General's Report on Mental Health*. www.surgeongeneral.gov/library/mentalhealth/home.html (accessed 3 October 2007).

Uzuhashi, T.K. (2001) Japan: bidding farewell to the welfare society, in P. Alcock and G. Craig (eds) *International Social Policy*. Houndmills: Palgrave, 104–23.

Vaithianathan, R. (2002) Will subsidising private health insurance help the public health system? *Economic Record*, 78: 277–83.

Walder, J. (2003) The USA approach to maternity care, *British Journal of Midwifery*, 11(8): 496–501.

Wall, A. and Owen, B. (1999) *Health Policy*. Sussex: Gildredge.

Wallace, W. (1997) *Why Vote Liberal Democrat?* Harmondsworth: Penguin.

Watts, D. (1994) *The Welfare State: A Suitable Case for Treatment*. Sheffield: Pavic Publications.

Webster, C. (1998) *The National Health Service: A Political History*. Oxford: Oxford University Press.

Webster, S. (2002) Voluntary action for health: a survey of the health benefits of the work of voluntary organisations in Leeds, in G. Morgan, D. Burns, G. Mountain, S. Pearson and M. Todd (eds) *Yorkshire Conference on Voluntary Sector Research 2002: Conference Proceedings*, part 2. Sheffield: Sheffield Hallam University Press.

Wells, J. (1995) Health care rationing: nursing perspectives, *Journal of Advanced Nursing*, 22: 738–44.

White House (2000) *The Clinton-Gore Administration: Working For A Strong, Enforceable Patients' Bill Of Rights*. Office of the Press Secretary. www.clinton4.nara. gov/WH/New/html/20000303.html (accessed 2 May 2008).

Whitehead, D. (2003) The health promoting nurse as a health policy career expert and entrepreneur, *Nurse Education Today*, 23: 585–92.

Whitehead, D. and Davis, P. (2001) The issue of medical dominance (hegemony), *Journal of Orthopaedic Nursing*, 5: 114–15.

Whitehead, M., Evandrou, M., Haglund, B. and Diderichsen, F. (1997) As the health divide widens in Sweden and Britain, what's happening to access to care?: Part 3, *British Medical Journal*, 315: 1006–9.

WHO (World Health Organisation) (1946) *Constitution of the World*. www.bradford. ac.uk/acad/sbtwc/btwc/int_inst/health_docs/WHO-CONSTITUTION.pdf (accessed 3 October 2007).

WHO (2003) *Organisation of Services for Mental Health: Mental Health Policy and Service Guidance Package*. www.who.int/bookorders/anglais/detart1.jsp?sesslan=1 &codlan=1&codcol=15&codcch=7543 (accessed 3 October 2007).

WHO (2004) *Mental Health Policy, Plans and Programmes*. www.who.int/entity/ mental_health/policy/en/policy_plans_revision.pdf (accessed 3 October 2007).

Wilding, K. (2002) Looking for clues: a practitioner perspective of third sector research in the UK, in G. Morgan, D. Burns, G. Mountain, S. Pearson and M. Todd (eds) *Yorkshire Conference on Voluntary Sector Research 2002: Conference Proceedings*, part 1. Sheffield: Sheffield Hallam University Press.

Wilkinson, G. and Miers, M. (1999) Power and professions, in G. Wilkinson and M. Miers (eds) *Power and Nursing Practice*. Houndmills: Macmillan.

Willems, S.J., Swinnen, W. and De Maeseneer, J.M. (2005) The GP's perception of poverty: a qualitative study, *Family Practice*, 22(2): 177–83.

Williams, A. (2000) *Nursing, Medicine and Primary Care*. Buckingham: Open University Press.

Wilson, A., Pearson, D. and Hassey, A. (2002) Barriers to developing the nurse practioner role in primary care – the GP perspective, *Family Practice*, 19(6): 641–6.

Winters, L., Gordon, U., Atherton, J. and Scott-Samuel, A. (2007) Developing public health nursing: barriers perceived by community nurses, *Public Health*, 121: 623–33.

Woodward, B. (2001) Confidentiality, consent and autonomy in the physician-patient relationship, *Health Care Analysis*, 9: 337–51.

Wuthnow, R. (1991) *Acts of Compassion: Caring for Others and Helping Ourselves*. Princeton: Princeton University Press.

Index